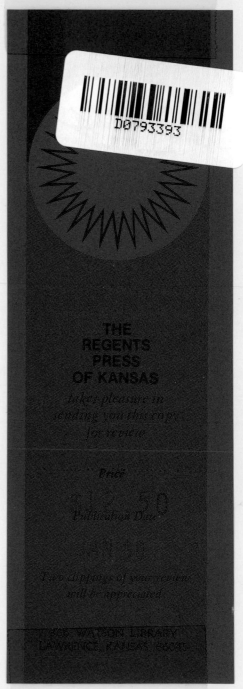

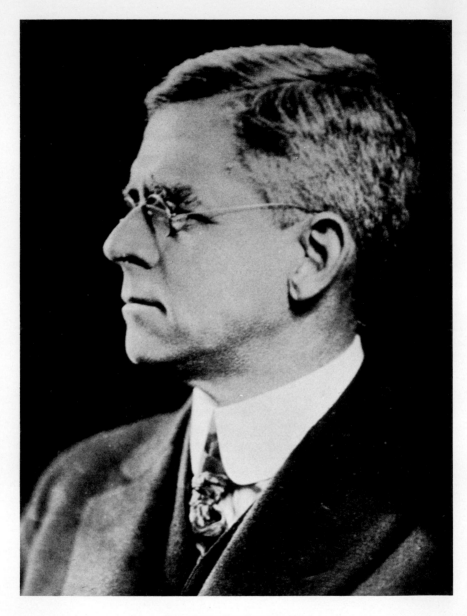

LUCIUS POLK BROWN
during the time of his employment in New York City

Courtesy of Susan Brown Lyon (Mrs. C. Hughes Lyon), Murfreesboro, Tennessee

LUCIUS POLK BROWN
AND
PROGRESSIVE
FOOD AND DRUG CONTROL

Tennessee and New York City
1908—1920

MARGARET RIPLEY WOLFE

THE REGENTS PRESS OF KANSAS
Lawrence

Library of Congress Cataloging in Publication Data

Wolfe, Margaret Ripley, 1947—
Lucius Polk Brown and progressive food and drug control.

Based on the author's thesis, University of Kentucky.
Bibliography: p.
Includes index.
1. Brown, Lucius Polk, 1867-1935. 2. Public
health personnel—United States—Biography.
3. Food adulteration and inspection—Tennessee—
History. 4. Drug adulteration—Tennessee—History.
5. Food adulteration and inspection—New York (City)
—History. 6. Drug adulteration—New York (City)—
History. 7. Progressivism (United States politics)
I. Title.
RA424.5.B76W64 1978   614.3'092'4 [B]   77-6637
ISBN 0-7006-0163-5

FOR

CLARENCE ESTILL
and
GERTRUDE BLESSING RIPLEY

Contents

Acknowledgments

I am indebted to many people for their contributions to this book. The following, however, have been particularly helpful. Dr. Frank B. Williams, chairman of the Department of History, East Tennessee State University, directed me to the subject of state food and drug control during the Progressive era when I was enrolled in his seminar on twentieth-century America. Another professor at that institution, Dr. Eric Russell Lacy, at the same time, whetted my interest in the process of professionalization. While I was engaged in doctoral study at the University of Kentucky, I wrote the dissertation on which this study is based. My special thanks go to Dr. Humbert S. Nelli, my major professor, whose excellent work served as an inspiration. I am grateful also to Dr. Richard Lowitt, whose enthusiasm and helpful suggestions were given freely throughout my residency. Professor John Duffy and the Russell Sage Foundation kindly allowed me to read portions of *A History of Public Health in New York City: 1866–1966* while it was being readied for publication. Professors Charles O. Jackson and James Harvey Young read the manuscript in its entirety and offered thoughtful, constructive criticism. Several librarians aided me in my research, but I must single out three individuals. Edith Keys, reference librarian at East Tennessee State University Sherrod Library, and Eloise Haney and Letitia Bullock, Kingsport University Center Library, were of inestimable assistance. My undying gratitude goes to the four children of Lucius Polk

Brown: Campbell Huxley Brown, Franklin, Tennessee; Susan Brown Lyon, Murfreesboro, Tennessee; Lizinka Brown Mosley, Nashville, Tennessee; and Lucia Brown Brownell, Birmingham, Alabama. All of them cooperated fully with my efforts to understand their father as a man and also the forces that motivated him in his work as a food and drug administrator. Susan Brown Lyon, a gracious southern lady, not only spent hours answering my numerous questions and searching for papers of her father's but also provided me with bed and board during my research trips.

Last of all, I express my appreciation to my husband David, who has had amazing forbearance in the face of short tempers and frayed nerves which naturally accompany scholarly work.

MARGARET RIPLEY WOLFE

Mt. Carmel, Tennessee

1—Introduction

From the 1890s to 1917 the United States thrashed about in a wave of reformism that originated and gained momentum in the urban centers, crested at the national level between 1900 and 1916, and ebbed with America's involvement in World War I. The feverishness of the times produced myriad political, social, economic, and scientific campaigns which met with some measure of success as well as numerous setbacks. One area of reform that has not received the attention to which it is entitled is the public health movement.[1] Specifically, state and municipal health matters of the Progressive era have been neglected by scholars. Nonetheless, the few existing studies deserve serious consideration.[2] Their coverage, however, leaves a great deal to the imagination when one tries to grasp the total picture of what municipal and state officials, as scientific people, encountered when they fought for the passage of new laws, struggled to enforce existing ones, and battled with the politicians, quacks, dissenting businessmen, and pervasive ignorance that threatened their efforts.

Thus, the field remains open for a comparative study of state and municipal health administration. For that purpose the career of Lucius Polk Brown serves as a vehicle to focus on food and drug work as one aspect of the public health movement within the context of Progressivism. In many respects Brown was typical of Progressive reformers. A middle-class, Anglo-Saxon Protestant and a professional, he represented a link between the nineteenth-century agrarian and

1

the twentieth-century urbanite. More importantly, however, such men as Brown in public life exhibited the features of a prototype, a new character on the American scene—a scientist out of the agricultural-experiment-station mold—ready to challenge politicians on their own ground, all in the name of reform. Major currents under way in American society affected the development of Brown's professional life and shaped his public career. The professionalization of science, the specialization of politics—varying in degree from North to South —and the tendency of reform efforts to spawn bureaucracies were significant forces acting on him.

Brown's entry into public life coincided with the professionalization of science and the peculiar specialization of politics. The rapid urbanization and industrialization of the late nineteenth century had spurred a drive toward professionalization. Trained specialists replaced the gentlemanly amateurs, formed exclusive organizations, and attempted to convince the public of their value to society. Autonomy—escape from outside control and regulation of the behavior of members—remained an elusive goal in American society.[3] Science and politics did not represent the only examples of the professionalization process, nor were they parallel in their development. These two areas of expertise are important to this study, however, because Brown, a professional scientist in government work, functioned in the same realm as professional politicians. The success of his work depended in large part on the degree of cooperation that could be achieved between the two rival power blocs. He, along with other scientists, required a favorable climate of opinion in securing funds to perpetuate his position and develop his ideas; politicians, too, curried the favor of the electorate in their never-ending search for votes. Because scientists and politicians found it imperative to operate in the same arena, their spheres of influence overlapped; and occasionally, scientists and politicians clashed when they became opponents struggling for autonomy.

As scientific knowledge, especially in bacteriology, grew in volume, public health reaped the benefits. Flamboyant reform crusades commonly occurred in cities. Brown's work as state pure food and drug inspector in Tennessee from 1908 to 1915 focused on cities and towns for practical reasons; his position as director of the Bureau of

Food and Drugs in the New York City Department of Health between 1915 and 1920 demanded specific concentration on urban problems. His presence and that of other scientists in the urban milieu alarmed politicians, not necessarily because their objectives differed, but because they jealously guarded their interests.

Cities not only fostered professional politicians and scientists but also served as their battlegrounds. In the cities the ward bosses and the urban machines they represented achieved a more cohesive organization than the political masters at any other level during the late 1800s and early 1900s. The careers of Martin Lomasney of Boston; "Big Tim" Sullivan, Richard Croker, and Charles F. Murphy—all of New York City; William Flinn of Pittsburgh; George B. Cox of Cincinnati; Roger B. Sullivan of Chicago; and Ed Crump of Memphis illustrated the adeptness of the urban bosses in the perfecting of professional techniques.[4]

The scientist, too, was an urban creature. Howard Mumford Jones, in *The Age of Energy*, has written: "The biological (or for that matter chemical or physical) laboratory is a creation of an urbanized culture. It requires lighting, heating, services of supply, continual sanitation, the aid of technicians, a capacity to acquire and install new instruments quickly, cold rooms, dark rooms, humidifiers, a continual supply of glassware, of specimens, of chemicals, of technical papers, all housed in a modern building which is theoretically possible on a country site but which in fact is seldom or never found very far away from an urban center."[5]

As urban characters, politicians and scientists developed their specialties. The professionalization that affected politicians in the post–Civil War generation resisted classification into such definite stages as that of science, but government service became a full-time occupation at the city, state, and national levels. As the population grew and the task of governing increased in complexity, American politics became the realm of a group of specialists who served an apprenticeship by performing menial party jobs. They collected rewards—patronage positions—for loyal service and graduated into an elite of highly skilled experts adept at the art of compromise.

Even contemporary observers noted the trend toward specialization that was taken by politics. Herbert Croly acknowledged that

3

politics, like business, had become specialized and organized when he proclaimed: "The American system of local self-government encouraged the creation of the political 'Boss,' because it required such an enormous amount of political business. Some one was needed to transact this business, and the professional politician was developed to supply the need."[6] Whitelaw Reid, editor of the *New York Tribune*, contended that governing the United States was an art that could not be learned in a week or two. Instead, the adroitness required to manage parties could be acquired only by long experience.[7] Social critic Lincoln Steffens, viewing politics as the realm of a special type of businessman rather than that of a professional politician, argued: "The politician is a businessman with a specialty. When a businessman of some other line learns the business of politics, he is a politician, and there is not much reform left in him. Consider the United States Senate, and believe me."[8]

The options of the politician varied, depending on his ambition and his ability. Municipalities afforded such nonelective posts as ward boss or chieftain of an urban machine. City government offered a number of elective possibilities as well. State offices had an attraction for some. The federal echelon served as a mecca for outstanding men in the field who scrambled for congressional posts and the juiciest political plum of all, the presidency. Whatever his goal, the expert conceived of himself as a professional whether he became a ward boss or reached the United States Senate.[9]

The gentlemanly reformer, unschooled in the art of politics, could expect little but scorn from the professional. George Washington Plunkitt, a district leader in the Tammany organization, vented his disgust with the inexperienced reform groups in the following manner: "They were mornin' glories—looked lovely in the mornin' and withered up in a short time, while the regular machines went on flourishin' forever, like fine old oaks." He further commented that the reformer could not sustain himself in politics because "politics is as much a regular business as the grocery or the dry-goods or the drug business. You've got to be trained up to it or you're sure to fail."[10] Such men as Plunkitt scorned all nonpolitical professionals in government, regardless of their credentials.

Professionalization was not isolated to the United States. Max

4

Weber, lecturing at Munich University in 1918, noted international trends toward professionalization and examined politics and science as they were developing in several Western countries. Overenthusiastically, he maintained that political bosses in the United States were "dilettantes" and that evils of such organizations as Tammany Hall could be eradicated by civil-service reforms. As for scientists, the sociologist implied that they should not become involved in politics or seek legitimation from outsiders. Their work, in itself, justified their existence.[11]

Weber's advice came too late for American scientists, who already were seeking recognition through various avenues including public service. Their course from amateurism to professionalization had proceeded systematically during the nineteenth century. They specialized, formed their societies, and received recognition as a legitimate elite. The alternatives for the professional scientist varied. Teaching, preferably at the university level, proved attractive for some; industry likewise had some allure. A few scientists chose self-employment in a consultative capacity. Government jobs, however, drew some of the most dynamic and politically oriented individuals.[12]

Lucius Polk Brown's experience in government service spanned twelve years and touched on two dissimilar political systems. Machine politics during the Progressive period were developed more thoroughly in the North than in the South. Although such urban bosses as Edward H. Crump of Memphis and such demagogues as Coleman L. Blease, Thomas E. Watson, and Benjamin R. Tillman could be found in the South, urban machines appeared more frequently in the North. The perfection of political strategy derived some motivation from the two-party system. Because the rural South during this time remained almost solidly Democratic as a consequence of the Civil War and its aftermath, the professionalization of politics was retarded.[13] Also, the absence of a substantial immigrant population and the fact that most Negroes in the South remained rural dwellers deprived would-be bosses of a natural following. The gentlemanly amateur still cropped up in southern state and local politics as a viable candidate of factions within a single party. In the North the gentlemanly amateur appeared but generally received the scorn of the professional, who looked on him for what he usually was, a reformer, "a mornin' glory."

5

Furthermore, the concentration of scientists appeared more frequently in large northern cities where greater opportunities existed. Scientists were scattered throughout the emerging urban areas south of the Mason-Dixon line; however, like their northern brethren, they felt the lure of government work. When the individual scientist entered the domain of the politician, he sometimes became a part of bureaucracies that were already in existence; or if he participated in reform crusades, he almost inevitably contributed to their creation. In doing so, he renounced much of his own freedom as a professional, tempering his own activities to fit the overall organizational purpose. Herein lay a potential area of conflict. The professional worker, closely aligned with his peers, was less likely to exhibit a high degree of loyalty to a particular organization than was a nonprofessional employee.[14] Brown waged his campaigns and fought his political battles as a professional scientist. Nevertheless, he sacrificed some of his professional independence when he entered the bureaucratic framework. His first experience in Tennessee did not call for abandonment of professionalism. Retention of the New York job after a political crisis in 1918 almost demanded that he forsake his identity as a scientist and complacently adjust to the role of a bureaucratic figurehead.

Lucius Polk Brown was a professional scientist who became a bureaucrat during an era when middle-class reformers first attempted to order American society through integrated systems. In Tennessee, he created an enforcement agency, enlarged its staff, developed a hierarchy of authority, and made it self-perpetuating. In New York City, he entered a metropolis with a maze of government agencies. The Department of Health alone had sufficient bureaus, administration, and staff to foster the inertia that was typical of latter-twentieth-century structures marked by excessive multiplication of power and concentration of authority.[15]

Brown's career provides a unique opportunity for studying a scientist involved in reform, evaluating his successes and failures within bureaucratic frameworks at different stages of development, and interpreting his struggles with politicians; it holds considerable potential for developing some fresh insights on the public health movement during the Progressive era. This book is first a study of a professional chemist who participated in food and drug control at the major governmental echelons—municipal, state, and federal. Second, it deals with Progressive health reform in the rural South and similar work in a northern metropolis. Third, it takes into consideration the accomplishments and failures of scientific experts who entered the realm of public health. Above all, however, it compares and contrasts the work of Brown within a developing bureaucracy in Tennessee and a well-established bureaucracy in New York City.

2—With Brown in Tennessee: The Right Man, the Right Place, the Right Time

As the twentieth century approached, Tennessee legislators and municipal authorities directed their attention to public health matters. Mindful of the health problems that had plagued generations of Americans and receptive to the scientific expertise that might alleviate these problems, lawmakers responded to the demands of concerned citizens. By 15 January 1908, when Governor Malcolm R. Patterson named Lucius Polk Brown to the post of state pure food and drug inspector, the state had a new law outlining his responsibilities and enough socially conscious residents to support his work. Brown's professional development had kept pace with the progress of public health in Tennessee. When the state needed someone with his qualifications, he was the right man, in the right place, at the right time.

Brown's heritage was Anglo-Saxon, Protestant, and southern agrarian. He was born at Hamilton Place in Maury County, Tennessee, on 1 April 1867—the oldest of the five children of George Campbell Brown and Susan Polk Brown. John Brown, the founder of the Brown family in the United States, was an Englishman who had come to America in the eighteenth century from Northern Ireland. A Presbyterian minister, he settled in Augusta County, Virginia, and established Liberty Hall Academy, the forerunner of Washington and Lee University. Lucius Polk Brown's great-grandfather, George Washington Campbell, became secretary of the treasury under President James

Madison, first minister of the delegation to Russia under President
James Monroe, and a senator from Tennessee; his grandfather, James
Percy Brown, served as an attaché to the American embassy in Paris.
His mother's people were the famous Polks of Middle Tennessee: his
great-grandfather, Colonel William Polk of Mecklenburg County,
North Carolina, fought in the Revolution; his great-uncle, Leonidas
Polk, was the Confederate general and Episcopalian bishop who had
once set out to make his fortune with a remedy for diphtheria; and
his cousin, James K. Polk, had been president of the United States.[1]

political family (handwritten margin note)

As a youth, Brown lived with his parents on Ewell Farm at Spring
Hill. He grew up during the difficult years of Reconstruction, but in
an atmosphere of gracious country living in the southern tradition.
He had the advantage of a sound preparatory education in private
schools, including Montgomery Bell Academy in Nashville and a high
school at Bellvue, Virginia. His family was not wealthy, but it was
financially secure because of its landholdings. The Browns had managed to retain more than eleven hundred acres when a wise executor
prevented the widow Elizabeth McKay Brown from investing in
Confederate bonds. In 1867 this same lady, by then the wife of General R. S. Ewell, brought the first registered Jersey cow to Tennessee.
Her interest in this particular breed contributed to the success of her
son Campbell as a stockbreeder and farmer and to the bent of her
grandson Lucius toward chemistry. As dairymen, the Browns placed
high priority on production standards, and chemical analysis held the
key for determining the quality of milk.[2]

Thus, Lucius Polk Brown turned toward chemistry. In the
autumn of 1885, when he was eighteen years old, he enrolled for his
first year of study at the University of Virginia. This signaled the
beginning of his preparation as a professional chemist. Instead of
pursuing a course of study that would have resulted in a professional
or titled academic degree, he earned untitled "degrees" in chemistry
and related sciences, an alternate program offered by the university
at that time. His college days, however, were not all spent in the
laboratory. The handsome, broad-shouldered, brown-eyed young man
also played football, rowed, and boxed. Professors acknowledged his
progress and recognized him as an able, conscientious student excel-
ling in laboratory courses.[3]

In 1889 Brown left the University of Virginia and returned to Tennessee. For the next four years he divided his time almost equally between farming and chemical experimentation in scientific agriculture. His contacts with agrarian life had remained open during his student days, for his father wrote to him often, informing him of activities at Ewell Farm and seeking his advice on the type of stock that should be purchased to improve the bloodlines of the dairy herd and the racehorses.[4]

Brown's return to the farm did not preclude his scientific interests; perhaps it promoted them, for he soon began laying foundations for his career as a chemist. In October 1889 he secured employment as acting chemist at the University of Tennessee Agricultural Experiment Station in Knoxville. Then in its infancy, the station itself had existed little more than two years, and the embryonic laboratory of the chemical division had been in operation only nine months when Brown became its director. His official duties included analysis of milk samples to determine butterfat content, comparison of varieties of sorghum to find the type best suited to the climate of Tennessee, and investigation of the quality of fertilizers.[5]

The pleasant interlude of professional work soon ended. Brown resigned as acting chemist with the experiment station, effective 1 July 1890, and returned to Ewell Farm to help his father, now aged and ill. Collecting samples from the herds of his prominent Middle Tennessee neighbors, the promising young chemist continued his work with methods for determining the content of butterfat in milk, especially those that could be adapted to the needs of the dairy farmer. He also kept himself informed of the results from similar tests at other state agricultural stations.[6] In 1893, Campbell Brown died, leaving Ewell Farm in the capable hands of his oldest son, who had been closely involved in operations there for the preceding three years. The responsibilities that Brown assumed left him little time for his chosen profession.

An ambitious man of varied interests and immense energy, Brown soon tired of the limited life of a farmer. Being an astute observer of contemporary events, he noted the rapid strides that the United States was making toward urbanization and industrialization. Neither he nor American society in the late nineteenth century could escape completely the rural heritage or resist the lure of urban dynamism. Now in his late twenties, he decided that the time had come to advance his career.

Nashville, in close proximity to Ewell Farm, became Brown's base of operation. Tennessee's largest city and capital boasted a population of 76,168 in 1890 and served as a major commercial and wholesale market between the Ohio River and the Gulf of Mexico. The pace of life in the city slowed during the depression of the 1890s, but in spite of economic difficulties, Nashvilleans could not have helped but notice the decisively urban qualities that their city reflected. The numerous buildings, the rapid suburban expansion, the business conducted, and the smoke billowing out of soft-coal furnaces legitimized claims of urbanization. Alongside the metropolitan features were holdovers from the less-sophisticated country town. Most of Nashville's inhabitants walked to work, to market, and to school; wealthier citizens had not yet fled the downtown area; and cows still grazed from 6 A.M. to 6 P.M. in certain designated places.[7]

To this town in transition, Brown went in search of opportunities as a professional chemist. By 1894 he had become a partner in the laboratory of Memminger & Brown, and eventually he assumed the ownership and presidency, changing the name to Lucius P. Brown & Company Analytical Chemists. From 1894 to 1908 his career advanced rapidly, and he established a reputation as an able chemist. Routine analysis consumed much of his time during these years, but his association with private companies provided him with other opportunities. For a time he served as director of both the Harley Pottery Company and the Hurricane Iron & Mining Company. His interest in geology and his involvement with these firms led to a number of mining ventures. He worked with phosphates in Tennessee and Florida over a period of several years, prospected for rutile in Virginia during 1903, and acquainted himself with the minerals of Utah, spending the summer of 1904 in that state.[8]

The aspiring professional at the turn of the century needed the approval of his peers. Graduate or advanced education, membership in professional organizations, and publication of articles and books offered the logical avenues to recognition. After Brown joined Memminger in Nashville, he continued his education at Vanderbilt University, where he enrolled as a graduate student in chemistry during 1897 and 1898. From 1894 to 1908 he joined such scientific organizations as the American Chemical Society and the Engineering Association of the South as well as a number of state and local societies. Later he affiliated with more highly specialized groups. He also published articles on the mining of phosphates in Tennessee, their quality, compositions, and uses.[9]

Changes in Brown's personal life accompanied his professional progress. In 1896 he was married to Jessie M. Roberts, the daughter of Albert Roberts, editor of the *Nashville American*. She died of pneumonia in 1897, leaving an infant son, Campbell Huxley. Brown remained a widower for six years. Then, in 1903, while on a prospecting trip in Virginia, he met Susan Catherine Massie, the sister of one of his classmates at the University of Virginia. They were married on 12 December 1903 at "Three Springs," the Massie home. The *Lynchburg News*, which carried a special article on the wedding, likened it to the "festive scenes of ante-bellum days." This union, which proved to be happy, produced three daughters, Susan Massie Polk, Lizinka Campbell, and Lucia Cabell.[10]

Toward the end of the 1890s a new sense of direction became evident in Brown's professional life. During earlier years he had dabbled in farming, agricultural chemistry, and private business. Increasingly, after the turn of the century, his orientation was toward government service. Keenly interested in the new pure food and drug campaign, he found opportunities awaiting him in the state government. On 14 January 1903, Brown applied to Governor James B. Frazier for formal recognition as chemist in the Tennessee Bureau of Agriculture. Because official occupants of that post had delegated their responsibilities to Brown over the years, he argued that his previous record showed his qualifications for the work. Apparently nothing came of the request, but Frazier asked him to represent Tennessee at a meeting of the National Association of State Dairy and Food Departments in St. Paul, Minnesota, in July. Brown did not show up at that meeting because he was in New York and did not receive the invitation in time, but when the eighth annual convention of food officials gathered at St. Louis in 1904, he attended. Thereafter, his career was intricately laced to this organization. His professional interests by this time definitely included government service as a specialist on food and drugs, and the annual meetings of the association provided forums for the exchange of ideas on legislation, enforcement, standards, and chemical procedures.[11]

By the time that Brown developed an affinity for food and drug control, efforts to improve public health had advanced tremendously. Social conscience and early modern scientific thinking had gradually supplanted demons, Divine Providence, and miasmas as explanations for disease. Although problems of gigantic proportion continued to haunt public health workers, beneficial changes were being made. By the late 1870s the germ theory had gained precedence over earlier views, largely as a consequence of the contributions made by the French chemist Louis Pasteur and Robert Koch, a German physician. Americans received this new knowledge with fascination and soon grasped its usefulness in the control of communicable diseases.[12]

Brown grew up in a state that was perplexed by typical health problems of the nineteenth century. Tennesseans reacted slowly but positively to new scientific discoveries. Their fears of recurring epidemics led to the establishment of the state and municipal boards of health. In Memphis, for example, the yellow-fever epidemic of 1878 had sparked improvements. Sanitary conditions there during Reconstruction resembled those of a medieval city. A pure water supply was practically nonexistent; unscrupulous dealers watered the milk they sold, polluting as well as diluting it. The *Public Ledger* of 18 September 1867 reported that the streets were "huge depots of filth, cavernous Augean stables, with no Tiber to flow through and cleanse them." Garbage, refuse, and dead animals produced a stench unrivaled, according to a carpetbagger, by that of Cairo and Cologne.[13]

When the epidemic of 1878 struck, most citizens fled, leaving behind a motley crew of Negroes, poor whites, self-appointed nurses and doctors, and some professional physicians. The horrors could be observed in decomposed human bodies and dead rats that had expired while eating diseased flesh. According to a medical estimate, the city lost 5,150 people out of a population that never exceeded 20,000 during the siege. The year after this catastrophe, officials established a public health program and a board to administer it.[14]

Memphis was not alone in its filth. Nashville was also notoriously unclean. Poorly drained streets, open sewers, and garbage heaps were commonplace. The privies, urinals, cesspools, and kitchen drains of the state penitentiary polluted streams that flowed through the town. Slaughterhouses discharged their offal in the same manner. Authorities there had first established a board of health in 1866, when Asiatic cholera appeared in the United States. The board floundered for a decade, however, until it came under the influence of John Berrien Lindsley. His work in Nashville, particularly during the yellow-fever epidemic of 1878, earned him the respect of the medical society. When in 1877 the Tennessee legislature created a state board of health in response to the demands of physicians, Lindsley became secretary; in 1884, president. The stinginess of the lawmakers hampered the work of the board; nevertheless, his efforts strengthened preventive medicine in the state.[15]

Health issues in Tennessee during the 1880s and 1890s continued to be relegated to the local level, and state administration remained weak. The most obvious interest in improvements came from health workers in the urban areas, but newspaper editors, writing for rural readers, frequently complained of unsanitary practices—if they could be attributed to the evils of city life. The editor of the *Clarksville Leaf-Chronicle* denounced the Nashville medical colleges for dumping barrels of dissected cadavers into the Cumberland River. In addition to creating sanitary problems, these strange cargoes washed up on river banks, presenting county coroners with numerous problems. Other state editors urged better care for the insane, denounced cigarette smoking, and opposed corsets and similar restrictive feminine apparel.[16]

Improvements in public health came slowly in Tennessee and elsewhere in the United States during the late nineteenth century. Rapid urbanization, mushrooming industrialization, and streams of immigrants complicated existing problems. The federal government made no move to interfere seriously with the practices of big business either in the realm of working conditions or in the quality of products manufactured. Without centralized control nationally, local governmental units could make little headway. Millions of immigrants from southern and eastern Europe flooded major industrial cities, serving as a ready supply of cheap labor for the factories. When accidents crippled them or they fell victims to diseases brought on by unfavorable working conditions and the abject poverty that low wages forced upon them, they became recipients of private charity or starved. Newcomers who maintained the strength to work congested the tenement districts and contributed to sanitary and housing problems. Cities were ill prepared to cope with the problems of the "new" immigrants. Even in New York City, where the Board of Health in 1866 had made such promising beginnings, political corruption and the overwhelming difficulties of the Lower East Side slowed the progress of public health.

The conditions of the streets, described by George Edwin Waring, Jr., as he found them in 1895 when he became director of the street-cleaning department, indicated that earlier efforts to purify New York City had been stymied:

> Rubbish of all kinds, garbage, and ashes lay neglected in the streets, and in the hot weather the city stank with the emanations of putrefying organic matter. It was not always possible to see the pavement, because of the dirt that covered it. One expert, a former contractor of street cleaning, told me that West Broadway could not be cleaned because it was so coated with grease from wagon axles; it was really coated with slimy mud. The sewer inlets were clogged with refuse; dirty paper was prevalent everywhere, and black rottenness was seen and smelt on every hand.[17]

Although such problems were not restricted to major metropolitan areas, their magnitude in large cities attracted attention. The reaction of socially conscious citizens to conditions of big-city life provided the impetus for Progressivism. Reality, to this generation of reformers, was "the bribe, the rebate, the bought franchise, the sale of adulterated food."[18] Wherever they found sordidness, neglect, or unpleasantness, whatever their motivations, they sought to change it. Once public health became an issue in this multifaceted campaign, it steadily increased in importance.

Pure food and drug control was in part an outgrowth of the "new" public health movement in urban areas, but it also owed its existence to agricultural scientists at the state experiment stations.

Although later in Brown's career he became aligned with big-city reformers, his first experience with food and drug purity and consumer protection stemmed from his brief tenure at the Tennessee Agricultural Experiment Station. During his years in private business, many of his counterparts continued to operate within the framework of experiment stations. As these bastions of scientific agriculture grew in importance, the work magnified in scope to include a concern for the purity of food, water, and drugs.[19]

The interest in food and drug control was well placed. As Walter Lippmann so aptly stated, the "ordinary purchaser" does not have time "to candle every egg he buys, test the milk, inquire into the origins of meat, analyze the canned food, distinguish the shoddy." Consumers were no better qualified to prescribe their own medicine. Yet, they stubbornly relied on the strange and exotic wares of patent-medicine dealers.[20]

Food and drug swindlers victimized the public, and state legislatures began passing laws designed to solve the problem. Often this occurred after legitimate businessmen urged the lawmakers to take action. These early efforts antedated the passage of effective food and drug laws to control the manufacture, distribution, and sale of products involved in interstate commerce. State officials soon recognized the need for federal regulation and launched a concerted effort to secure congressional approval. They were aided by the revelations of such muckrakers as Samuel Hopkins Adams and Upton Sinclair. Adams exposed the evils of patent medicines and related malpractices in his series "The Great American Fraud," printed in Collier's Weekly. Upton Sinclair, a foremost critic of American society, attempted to win converts to socialism with The Jungle, but readers bogged down in the gory, nauseating descriptions of the Chicago meat-packing industry.

Concern for a better quality of food was not limited to muckrakers and local officials. After the Spanish-American War, General Nelson A. Miles raised a cry against impure food when he charged that "embalmed beef" had caused sickness among soldiers in Cuba. In May 1903, Dr. Harvey W. Wiley, chief chemist of the Department of Agriculture, organized his famous "poison squad" to determine the effects that artificial additives in foods had on the human body.

The findings indicated that all such substances were deleterious, a position that Wiley doggedly maintained throughout his career.[21]

Although sensationalism was important in securing the passage of national legislation, the careful behind-the-scenes efforts of the Association of State and National Food and Dairy Departments proved to be the determining factor. As early as August 1897 these scientific reformers, many of whom were cast in the experiment-station mold, came together at Detroit for the first annual convention. From this time until 1906 they waged a relentless campaign to promote passage of federal regulation. No less a person than President Theodore Roosevelt recognized the role played by state food and dairy inspectors. In a message to Congress, Roosevelt made these remarks: "It is primarily to the action of these State commissioners that we owe the enactment of this law, for they aroused the people, first to demand the enactment and enforcement of State laws on the subject, and then the enactment of the Federal law without which the State laws were largely ineffective."[22]

With the passage of the Pure Food and Drug Law of 1906, most states updated their statutes to complement the federal legislation. Those having no enforcement apparatus moved to establish some agency for food and drug control. Brown's native state had given little support to the battle for domestic food and drug legislation at the national level, but Tennessee lawmakers could not totally ignore the Progressive forces at work in the nation. In 1897 they reorganized the state Board of Health. Consisting of three physicians and the state commissioner of agriculture, as ex officio member, the new board numbered among its duties the responsibility for enforcement of the pure food laws. The effrontery of the legislature at this time could hardly be exaggerated. While authorizing the board to establish and equip a chemical and biological laboratory "with such experts as they may elect," the lawmakers emphasized: "It is the duty of said board to see that the provisions of this act are carried out without any additional appropriations."[23]

Genial Democratic Governor Robert L. Taylor, in his biennial message of 1899, reminded the legislature of its obligations: "We have a pure food law as many other states have. Other states are putting their laws into execution, and therefore driving the adulterers and dealers in impure food into states which have no such laws, or if they have them, they are not executing them. We are in the condition of having the law on our statute books with no appropriation for its execution." The governor then recommended: "In the interest of the producers and for the consumers of our state, I suggest that your honorable bodies would do well to confer with the members of the Board of Health upon this important question, and act and make such appropriation as you may feel the best interest of the state requires."[24] Four successive legislatures, however, made no concrete efforts to implement the enforcement of existing laws.

In the Fifty-first General Assembly of 1899, proposals dealing with the regulation of the sale of narcotics and impure food died in the House Committee on Sanitation. In 1901, new bills met the same fate, with the exception of legislation to empower the state Board of Health to enforce the pure food law; the Committee on Sanitation recommended passage, but no further action was taken. A bill to prevent adulteration of food and beverages, sponsored by John Watson Morton of Davidson County, came to a vote on the floors of both houses in 1903. The House favored it 56 to 28, but the Senate rejected it 17 to 9. The legislators of 1905 saw no measures come to a vote in both houses.[25]

Voting patterns from 1899 to 1905 revealed no obvious opposition bloc to food and drug legislation, although Republicans from East Tennessee and a few Democrats from Shelby and Knox counties sometimes voted negatively. On the other hand, delegates from the same areas occasionally cast positive votes. Of the four major urban areas—which included Knoxville, Chattanooga, Nashville, and Memphis—the representatives from Davidson County and Nashville most consistently lent their support; those from Memphis and Shelby counties, their opposition. The intransigence of the legislature apparently was not a product of any carefully conceived plan to prevent passage of pure food and drug bills but, rather, the failure of the representatives and senators to take upon themselves the responsibility for additional appropriations. In all likelihood, the legislature, consisting primarily of representatives from rural areas, believed that the cities, where the exchange of most goods took place, should assume the burden of maintaining food and drug purity.

Before the Fifty-fifth General Assembly convened in 1907, Congress had enacted national legislation. The federal law that was signed on 30 June 1906 applied to the manufacture, sale, or transportation of adulterated, misbranded, poisonous, or deleterious foods, drugs, medicines, and liquors. This law, however, was limited to the manufacture of such items in the territories and the District of Columbia, and it applied to interstate traffic. If a state failed to enact and enforce laws of its own, unscrupulous and ignorant dealers were at liberty to manufacture and distribute dangerous goods within its boundaries. The recent federal action and the responsibilities it placed on the states themselves for their internal safety from adulterated food and drugs, coupled with pressure from concerned citizens, finally moved the Tennessee legislature.[26]

The debate over the pure food and drug issue in 1907 centered on two questions: (1) whether to enact a new law or make an appropriation to enforce the old one; and (2) if a new law were passed, to whom responsibility for enforcement should be assigned. Shortly after the legislature convened in January, Representative Currie Dixon of Haywood County announced that he would try to secure sufficient appropriation to enforce the pure food law of 1897. He estimated the cost at a modest $3,000 per annum. This move was accompanied by a statement from medical authorities that the amount of food adulteration in Tennessee was "something startling." Within a week, two bills were introduced in the General Assembly to prevent the manufacture of adulterated food and drugs, one assigning responsibility for enforcement to the Board of Health and the other creating a new office. Another measure required manufacturers of patent medicines to list the ingredients of their products on the labels.[27]

Sponsored by Democrat W. B. Marr of Davidson County, House Bill 141, discarding the old law and calling for creation of a new office, showed the most promise. Governor Malcolm R. Patterson supported the concept of a separate office. In his address to the legislature on 23 January, he called the food and drug law of 1897 "practically a dead letter," and he urged that it be revitalized by an appropriation or that a new one similar to the national act be passed. He further recommended the creation of the office of state chemist, "to be filled by a man of established reputation in his profession," and that this official be responsible for enforcement of the food and drug laws.[28]

Even with executive support, Marr's bill did not pass before it had been carefully scrutinized by legislative committees, the Board of Health, businessmen, pharmacists, physicians, and farmers. When the House Committee on Sanitation met, members of the medical profession, merchants, and manufacturers appeared to debate the merits of the measure. The committee attached an amendment to the bill, which provided that it should take effect on 1 January 1908, and unanimously recommended it for passage. Shortly after this action, on 4 February, the Board of Health called a special meeting to consider all pending health measures, including those dealing with food and drugs; but they took no action. Druggists from Nashville and other cities met the next day at the headquarters of the local board of trade. They decided to do whatever was necessary to protect their own interests, an indication that they were not completely favorable to the pending legislation. The House Committee on Finance, Ways and Means held two long sessions before approving the bill. In the interim, "some unknown party," according to the sponsor of the bill and other irate lawmakers, took the document out of chambers and changed it materially. At the second meeting of the finance committee, the measure generated a heated discussion, then squeaked through by a vote of 9 to 7. While committees debated and stalled, farm organizations and medical societies urged passage. When the bill finally came to a vote in the House, representatives approved it by a vote of 74 to 19.[29]

The Marr bill encountered difficulties in the Senate Committee on Finance. Druggists were on hand to present their views. Their representative, Charles Martin, urged that the state law conform as nearly as possible to the federal act and that responsibility for its enforcement be entrusted to a commission made up of the secretary from the Board of Health, the commissioner of agriculture, and the secretary of the State Board of Pharmacy. The finance committee recommended that a druggist be placed on the Board of Health and that a Senate measure known as the Mansfield bill be substituted for the Marr bill. When the issue came before the full Senate, they debated how enforcement should be handled. Interestingly enough, both the Senate and the House largely ignored the position of pure food and drug inspector, proposed by the Marr bill. The idea that enforcement belonged with the Board of Health instead of with "men who have interest in its non-enforcement" prevailed in the Senate. The Mansfield measure was tabled, and the Marr bill was called up for a vote. The Senate approved it, 21 to 9, and sent it to the governor. Patterson signed it on 9 April.[30]

The new Pure Food and Drug Act of 1907 complemented federal legislation. Under its provisions, no person could "manufacture for sale, produce for sale, have in possession with intent to sell, or sell or give away, any article of food and drugs" that was adulterated or misbranded. Violation was a misdemeanor. Conviction for the first offense carried a fine of not less than $10 or more than $100, ninety days' imprisonment in the county jail, or both; a second offense, not less than $100 or more than $1,000, imprisonment for not more than eleven months and twenty-nine days, or both. To enforce this law, the General Assembly created the position of pure food and drug inspector, to be filled by "a chemist of established reputation and ability," chosen by the governor for a term of two years beginning 15 January of the year appointed; his salary was to be $2,500 a year. Responsibilities included the establishment and maintenance of an office and laboratory and the inspection and analysis of food and drug samples. To accomplish these objectives, the inspector received $1,000 "or as much thereof as may be necessary" per year, not to exceed $100 a month. The law required that he keep careful expense accounts, report to the Board of Health as often as requested and to the governor annually, and publish all violations at least twice a year.[31]

Because Lucius Polk Brown's varied experience in chemistry qualified him for the office of pure food and drug inspector, he followed legislative action on the Marr bill with considerable interest. Securing appointment, however, required careful political maneuvering. Even as Patterson considered the matter, local opposition to state and national food and drug legislation mounted. Early in 1908 the quality of food and drugs in Tennessee was as unacceptable as in the rest of the nation. Amid rumors of stringent federal enforcement, A. M. Tillman, a district attorney in Nashville, declared that a product branded "strawberry jelly" was as likely to be turnips as anything else. Wholesale grocers, according to Tillman, did not like the food and drug legislation because they found it humiliating to depreciate their products with revealing labels. One Nashville grocer, fearing federal enforcement and presaging future difficulties, reported that the local courts would impose only minimum fines; he did not know what the recourse would be if the federals moved into the city.[32]

With opposition already in evidence, the governor selected his appointee with care. The office of pure food and drug inspector carried a relatively substantial salary and held enormous possibilities for political favoritism. As soon as the law went into effect, Brown mobilized his supporters. On 2 January he conversed with John Thompson, the secretary of agriculture, who volunteered to talk to the governor on his behalf. The secretary, nevertheless, believed that politics required the appointment of a man from Memphis. That same day the applicant also saw Dr. S. S. Crockett and suggested that he use Thompson to convey to Patterson the endorsement of the medical profession and to refer to the advantages of selecting someone with a private laboratory, because the legislature had not appropriated enough money to equip such a facility. Brown's candidacy received a considerable boost, a few days later, when the Board of Health and Representative Marr endorsed him.[33]

Patterson called Brown to the capitol on 9 January for an interview and asked him to return two days later, at which time he informed him that he thought his appointment possible. While making suggestions concerning the work of the new department, Patterson emphasized its importance to his administration. Although the inspector was to ignore politics as much as possible, the chief executive made it clear that he expected support from all of his appointees. Brown assured the governor that he would give both political and personal devotion, and Patterson promised to make the official announcement on 15 January 1908. Fortunately, Brown, a Democrat, never found it difficult to keep his commitment, for throughout the years that he worked as a food and drug administrator he came to respect and like Patterson for his intelligence and sense of fairness.[34]

A combination of forces had led to enactment of the state pure food and drug law and the appointment of Lucius Polk Brown to the post of pure food and drug inspector. These included an increase in scientific knowledge; the intensification of environmental problems by urbanization and industrialization, which sparked Progressivism and gave new impetus to public health reform; the mobilization of muckrakers, agricultural scientists, and other groups that crusaded for federal regulation of food and drugs; and Brown's professional interests, which steered him toward food and drug control and consumer protection.

In 1907, state legislators seemingly acknowledged the soundness of scientific theory and succumbed to reform propaganda. Their almost innate financial conservatism had not been eradicated, however, by the mere enactment of a law. Their miserly habits revealed themselves in the small appropriation. Nonetheless, Lucius Polk Brown knew their ways and their limitations and sought opportunities to expand his department and increase its effectiveness. Once the quest for pure food and drugs had begun, it dominated health matters in Tennessee for almost eight years. The flamboyant crusade owed its success and its prominence to Brown, whose personality and character determined the course to be followed in building a bureaucracy and enforcing the law.

3—The Scientist
as a Southern Bureaucrat, 1908-11

Tennessee, at the turn of the century, was a slow-moving southern state. Prohibition, feminist agitation, and communal living commanded the attention of a few, but most residents conducted their lives in a leisurely, simple fashion. Occasionally, the Democratic party, which represented the overwhelming majority of Tennesseans, suffered from factionalism; but in 1897, Robert Love Taylor returned to the governor's chair, and dissidence subsided temporarily. The nineteenth century in the state closed with a centennial extravaganza. Preparations remained incomplete in 1896 when the one-hundredth anniversary of statehood occurred, but residents celebrated unabashedly the next year. Fights over the liquor question, however, punctuated the early years of the twentieth century, disrupting the relative tranquility of the state.[1]

When Lucius Polk Brown became pure food and drug inspector in Tennessee, a dynamic individual entered a social and political environment that was about to be torn by prohibition. This issue dominated state politics during the first two decades of the twentieth century. Brown, however, attracted support for pure food and drug control, an important side issue, and, at the same time, remained aloof from the political squabbles brought on by the liquor question. This feat, lasting from 1908 to 1911, was made possible by the nature of Tennesseans. Not the type, generally, to seek out new ideas, they waited for floods of national reform to wash over them. They were cautious in their thinking and were often suspicious of outsiders. As a native, Brown possessed definite advantages. He had distinguished ancestors in a society that placed importance on such matters, and he came from a prominent farming family. His ties to the soil, in a state composed of 1,743,744 rural dwellers in a total population numbering no more than 2,184,789 in 1910, earned him the respect of an agrarian people. While they might believe some of his ideas strange, they did not reject them outright.[2]

Acceptance as an individual was one matter; developing and enforcing a successful food and drug control program, another. In Tennessee, Brown faced problems that ran the full gamut—mislabeling and adulteration by design and ignorance, malicious intent to cheat customers, and drug addiction were commonplace. Ignorance posed a more serious threat than malice. Although Brown was an able chemist, food and drug administration was a new field for him. Furthermore, he faced the responsibility of establishing an entirely new department in the state government.

Between 1908 and 1911 Brown's inexperience, combined with the problems inherent in the establishment of a government agency, gave the appearance of confusion as he groped for policy and pleaded for additional financial assistance. Out of the chaos, however, he gradually built an enforcement agency that was acceptable to the majority of Tennesseans. More of a practical scientist than an ivory-tower philosopher, Brown kept his ideas simple. A realist, he knew that his work depended on public approval. He therefore devoted considerable time to selling the concept of food and drug control, and he moved cautiously against businessmen who violated the law. He believed that proper public health education, coupled with fair enforcement of the laws, would provide the remedy for Tennessee's problems. His first two terms in office were formative ones for him as well as his department. His enforcement was sketchy and fragmented as he uncovered the varied difficulties of food and drug control in the state, but during this time he gained valuable experience and improved the quality of goods available to consumers.

Brown began building an enforcement agency as soon as he was appointed. The development of this office from 1908 to 1915 demonstrated the remarkable tendency of Progressive innovations in government to become expansive. During his tenure, Brown obtained departmental status for his office; changed his title from inspector to commissioner, in fact if not in law; enlarged the investigative force from a one-man operation to an eight-man agency directly involved with inspection; and secured increases in appropriations, which raised them from $4,700 in 1908 to more than $25,000 in 1914.[3]

TENNESSEE PURE FOOD AND DRUG DEPARTMENT IN 1908

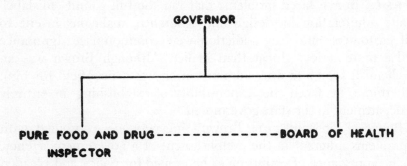

Although these alterations in the potential of the food and drug department were dramatic, they hardly kept pace with the new responsibilities being assigned to it, some of which were actively encouraged by Brown. A report authorized by the Council on Health and Public Instruction of the American Medical Association contained a thumbnail sketch of the Tennessee department as it appeared in 1915, the year that Brown left the state to assume a new position in New York City:

> The department of food and drugs is supposed to be under the supervision of the department of health, but the connection is slight, as the chief inspector is appointed directly by the governor, and there is a special appropriation for the department. Six inspectors and two chemists are supposed not only to look after adulteration, including milk, but to enforce the "sanitary law" in regard to the cleanliness of hotels, restaurants, bakeries, stores, slaughterhouses, etc., the "hotel law," and the very important "anti-narcotic law," as

well as to assist in the enforcement of the "weights and measures" law. Nevertheless, good work has been done by this small force.[4]

This description indicated that the office of pure food and drug inspector carried substantial possibilities for political favoritism. The Board of Health exerted some influence over the inspector, for the law required that he make periodic reports whenever the board might request them; he reported to the governor only once a year. He, therefore, determined standards of purity, sanitation, and quality with almost no direct supervision. Although the Board of Health had some control, the Food and Drug Department, as it evolved under Brown, took the initiative and received full cooperation and no opposition from that agency. Thus, no system of checks or balances really affected the inspector except the likelihood that the governor would not reappoint him when his two-year term expired if his policies had been politically detrimental to the administration.

The Tennessee legislators had created opportunities for scientific tyranny which could have been seized upon by an unscrupulous appointee if the governor had made a poor choice. The majority of the lawmakers were probably as unconcerned about this remote possibility as the National Association of State Dairy and Food Departments had been in 1902 when the issue had been raised. An editorial from a western newspaper, read at the annual convention by Dr. William C. Mitchell of the Colorado State Board of Health, commented on "a dangerous tendency toward a centralization of power" to be found in a certain provision of the Hepburn pure food bill. The proposed legislation made the chief chemist of the Department of Agriculture the sole judge of food and drug standards, which the editorial deemed "a power more absolute and quite as far reaching as any ever enjoyed by the most absolute of monarchs and one which would raise visions of opportunities for 'grafting' so stupendous as fairly to stagger the imagination of even the most ambitious of 'political bosses.' "[5]

The thinking of the experts who urged passage of the food and drug legislation and of the lawmakers who responded to them provided an example of the myopia that characterized the Progressive generation. The experts pitted themselves, as the champions of society, against evil food and drug adulterators, but they ignored or failed to realize the possibilities for usurpation of individual freedom that were at their disposal. They drafted legislation creating jobs for themselves; secured the appointment of each other through professional recommendations; banded together in national, state, and regional organizations; and enforced, largely at their own discretion, the laws that they helped to write. To their credit, it should be noted that most of these people were conscientious, public-spirited officials who tried to educate those who were affected by the laws and to prosecute them only as a last resort.

In Tennessee, Brown steered a moderate course although opportunities abounded for political favoritism and unreasonable standards. The situation in which he found himself at the time of his appointment could only be described as bewildering for the most dedicated official. Given the absence of an effective state health administration, it would not have been surprising if he had taken on dictatorial tendencies. Brown, however, calmly set about almost immediately organizing the work of his one-man department and developing strategy for a crusade against impure food and drugs. The speedy establishment of a laboratory to test samples was an absolute necessity for effective enforcement. Inadequate funds prevented him from setting up an independent state laboratory. He owned private facilities, however, located at 818 Church Street in Nashville, a godsend for the state and probably a factor in his appointment. The Board of Health directed him to purchase additional equipment and to put aside two rooms in his building for state work; no sublaboratories existed. Eventually, the department moved to offices in the capitol annex.[6]

Brown was as concerned about preparing himself for his new duties as he was with organizing his department and informing the public. To feel sure of himself and his interpretation of the state law, he requested a meeting with Charles T. Cates, Jr., the state attorney general. When they discussed legal matters on 19 February 1908, they found themselves essentially in agreement. To keep abreast of national developments, Brown established close ties with Harvey W. Wiley and the various organizations of food officials. Within three weeks of his appointment, the inspector went to Washington, D.C., to discuss with Wiley the correlation of state and national investigation of food and drugs. The *Nashville Banner* carried an overly optimistic report of the trip as well as the preliminary work of the new appointee. According to the newspaper, everything necessary to begin work had been established, and enforcement of the state law would begin immediately. Brown, a man not given to overstatement, recorded in his diary that the comments were "entirely unwarranted."[7]

After setting up an office and acquainting himself with the law, Brown initiated a program to inform the public of the dangers presented by adulterated food and drugs. A concerned citizenry, as he knew, could exert enough pressure to force state legislators to fund the department adequately. While touring the cities and towns of Tennessee in search of impure food and drugs, the inspector lectured. Described as not having been an "after-dinner speaker," he wasted little time on formalities. He focused his attention on common problems, how they could affect human health, and how they should be remedied. His itinerary of October 1908 included stops in Crossville, Lafollette, and Chattanooga as well as the Nashville area. In Chattanooga he collected samples and talked with a group of physicians, an effort that Brown described as "only moderately successful."[8]

In the beginning he was confined largely to Nashville and to Davidson County because of limited resources. As money and help increased, so did the scope of investigation and enforcement. Nonetheless, Brown covered a good deal of territory, even in 1908. In December he spoke again in Chattanooga, this time to the Kosmos Club. He complimented them on their city market, talked about his work, and used stereopticon slides to illustrate his lecture. Later, one city physician told the club the reason that their city had no inspector: "There are five good reasons," he said, "the mayor and four commissioners."[9] The apathy of local officials, however, could not deter interested citizens. By 1909 Chattanooga had a market inspector.

Aware of the attitude of dishonest businessmen toward adverse publicity and informed customers, the framers of the state pure food and drug law had provided for the publication of the names of offenders. In Brown's first report to the Board of Health, he outlined plans for issuing bulletins dealing with misbranding and adulteration. He tried, however, to give businessmen every opportunity to conform to the law before subjecting them to prosecution. Shortly after his appointment, he conferred with the Board of Pharmacists, whose members promised their assistance and requested fair treatment. In an effort to enlighten the merchants of Nashville, he addressed the Retail Grocers and Merchants' Association in mid March. A Nashville newspaper reported that a unanimous resolution favoring the state law had been adopted at the meeting. Joseph Ezell, president of the group, in a letter to the editor, declared that the article was incorrect: "It has been reported in your paper of the 17th that the Retail Grocers and Merchants' Association at their meeting Monday night passed a resolution endorsing the state pure food law. This is a mistake which we desire to correct, as no such resolution was even introduced at the meeting."[10]

The rebuttal had its significance. Not all members of the local trade association supported the law or the inspector. Resentment festered, but the political climate was not favorably disposed toward the businessmen until late in 1911. The state pure food and drug law, however, remained a topic of conversation at their meetings. In February 1909, H. L. Scott, a grocer, proposed that the law be amended to conform to national standards.[11] Apparently those who participated in the discussion remained ignorant of their foe, for this act was merely an extension of national legislation. Their comments reflected their apprehension; members of the association had not yet decided whether to submit to the authority of the pure food and drug inspector.

The suspicions of the food dealers were unwarranted, for Brown dealt fairly with businessmen. Following the course outlined in the Pure Food and Drug Law, he took samples from food and drugs believed to be adulterated, analyzed them, and issued warnings which were followed by prosecutions if a second sample showed that the dealer had failed to comply with standards. During his first year in office, he issued three circulars. The first summarized the Pure Food and Drug Act; the second described the minimum standards for syrups and molasses, which he put into effect on 1 October; and the third, addressed to those selling food and drinks at fairs and other public gatherings, dealt with sanitary procedures.[12] Any food dealer who openly opposed the law placed himself in a precarious situation, for he invariably alienated some of his customers; a few businessmen took the risk. The inspector, in late 1908, said that some merchants regarded pure food laws as interference with their "inalienable rights." He emphasized that he was concerned only with common honesty and the health of the people.[13]

To give merchants and manufacturers ample opportunity to conform, Brown made no hurried attempt to enforce the law strictly during 1908. By late October, however, he had misgivings about his policy when he discovered, while on a tour of the state, that merchants, although warned of the consequences, flagrantly violated the law. He reminded them that a second offense would result in prosecution.[14] If his findings, based on the examination of 517 samples collected from April 1908 to January 1909, were indicative of the quality of food and drugs for the state as a whole, clearly a great need existed for the rigid enforcement of the statutes; 53.17 percent were illegal or adulterated.[15]

Realizing the nature of human beings as well as the grave consequences that impure products had on the health of the public, Brown tried to maintain his keen sense of humor in dealing with' jobbers, merchants, and patent-medicine men. Early in 1908 he entered into a lively discussion with a dealer in sugar cakes who had marked his cakes "Home Made." Brown insisted that this title be removed from the label because the product resembled maple sugar. Later in the year he encountered a patent-medicine man who sold a remedy called Lethia. The inspector decided that the label was not legitimate, the product having been named for the mythical Greek river of Lethe in Hades, whose water, when consumed, caused forgetfulness. The official himself was often the butt of jokes, which he took in stride. He found a letter from a friend of his brother George's particularly amusing. It arrived in a peculiar envelope bearing an advertisement for Red Raven Splits, a soda water. Labeled in large red letters, it proclaimed: "Joe Anderson, The Live Druggist, Chattanooga to Lucius Polk Brown, Meddler, Deviler, Fly Inspector, Pure Food and Other People's Business."[16]

While some of the labels were amusing, others misled and cheated customers. Grocers, for example, willfully or unwillfully, robbed their customers by selling oysters containing an illegal content of water.

During January and February 1909, Nashvilleans consumed 30,000 quarts of oysters. If these contained 35 percent more water than was legal, something that was not unusual, then approximately 10,500 quarts of water were sold as oysters. Assuming that merchants sold the seafood at 35 cents a quart, customers paid $3,675 for water.[17]

By the end of Brown's first year in office, Tennesseans began to realize the value of pure food and drug regulation. Newspapers had given complimentary coverage throughout 1908. Not until late in the year, however, did organizations praise Brown publicly, indicating that a strong base of support was developing for him and his work. The Nashville Housekeepers' Club passed a unanimous resolution endorsing his actions. Likewise, the Nashville Board of Trade commended him and approved his ruling that hotels, restaurants, cafés, boarding houses, and all public places where meals were served should inform their patrons as to whether they served butter or oleomargarine.[18]

Brown's first year as pure food and drug inspector proved to be a crucial one, for it provided him the time that he needed to begin public health education, establish a fledgling department, attract staunch supporters, and alert office seekers to the political potential of his work. Furthermore, he found it desirable to coordinate his goals with those of other food and drug officials at the state and federal levels. The lessons he learned during 1908 made it possible for him to conceive of a logical course of action for the future. From 1909 to 1915 his activities centered on four major objectives: waging campaigns against those who were violating the laws, educating the masses to public health needs, increasing the size and power of his department, and building a national reputation for himself in his profession. Frequently these objectives blurred and overlapped, but they represented the basis of his operations. Although hampered by limited funds, his work remained relatively undisturbed by mounting political tensions in the state until the latter part of 1911. During the intervening years, Brown established a department capable of weathering the storm that could have wrecked it, developed a general philosophy of enforcement, and built a reputation for himself that was impervious to petty political attacks.

Brown's initial efforts suited politicians and other state bureaucrats, paving the way for additional legislation to promote his work. Early in 1909, Representatives Samuel Lee Chesnutt, representing Hawkins and Sullivan counties, and David B. Puryear of Sumner County introduced a bill in the House, requiring sanitary conditions in all places where food was prepared, manufactured, packed, stored, or distributed. Written by the Association of State and National Food and Dairy Inspectors, recommended by Brown, and supported by the governor, this legislation, complementing that of 1907, passed without any difficulty.[19] The Board of Health rallied wholeheartedly to back Brown during his first year, and when it met in May 1909, it authorized the inspector to appoint deputies to help him enforce the Sanitary Food Law. The health authorities also commended the legislature for having provided funds to add an assistant chemist to the Pure Food and Drug Department.[20]

In the same year, Democratic Senator J. T. Baskerville sponsored a bill to "prevent fraud in the weights of articles" sold in the state. Although the measure was weakly constructed, it passed, and it helped Brown to cope with mislabeling. Subsequently, when the inspector became an official of the Bureau of Weights and Measures of the United States, he requested and received authority to take charge of the standard weights and measures located in the state capitol and to act as state sealer. He declared that the creation of a separate bureau would be unnecessarily expensive.[21]

This tactic of voluntarily taking on additional responsibilities or of making recommendations that would lead to other duties resulted by 1915 in a significant accumulation of power in the hands of one man. Acting often on Brown's recommendations, the legislature made the Pure Food and Drug Department a catchall for miscellaneous chores requiring some scientific expertise. As its duties increased, the department grew stronger and gained a degree of security. Certainly the prerogative of the inspector to prosecute could have been used maliciously, but Brown used the power of enforcement sparingly. After ample time had been provided for food suppliers to conform with the existing legal standards, he adopted a method that was common among Progressive reformers for dealing with flagrant offenders. He put his technique—the campaign—into effect during the summer of 1909 and revived it thereafter when the need arose, usually during the sultry months of spring and summer. The characteristics of the campaign technique included a full-scale inspection of a given city or town for a period of time that generally ranged over a week or two. Accompanied by officers from his own department, when they became available, by city and county health officials, and by newspaper reporters, the pure food and drug inspector descended on food-handling establishments. When he discovered dealers who violated the law, he subjected them to the righteous indignation of the press, but infrequently to prosecutions and fines.

The summer campaign of 1909 in Nashville had all the trappings of those that were to follow. On 11 May, Brown swept down on the lawbreakers like an avenging angel. He received full local press coverage, wreaking undesired publicity on the offenders. Concerning himself especially with contamination by the common housefly, he staunchly avowed: "I will continue the campaign until the whole city is in good shape." Fifty places were inspected the first day at the city market. Brown found that there were numerous violations, and he issued orders demanding full compliance with legal standards. One of the greatest needs proved to be screened windows and doors. Alluding to the Sanitary Food Law, which had become effective on 1 May, the inspector declared: "An ounce of prevention is worth a pound of cure." He stated that he had encountered little opposition because ignorance, not indifference, was his greatest foe; and he occasionally referred to another proverb when he dealt with lawbreakers: "Cleanliness is next to Godliness."[22] Brown indulged in these platitudes because they could be understood by the lawbreakers and the general public.

Two days later, Brown—accompanied by Blaine Dudley, the inspector of food and marketing in Nashville, and a reporter from the *Banner*—toured the city, inspecting stores. They found unscreened windows and doors, toilets adjoining kitchens, open jars of refuse, dirty walls, dusty bread trays, an absence of cuspidors, and decaying food. Flies and insects entered easily from all sides. Chickens roamed freely in one establishment. Wherever the inspector went, owners generally received him with courtesy—tainted by a degree of distrust.[23]

Efforts in Nashville continued throughout the summer. In July,

Brown issued an ultimatum that the farmers' market must be screened by the end of the month. Twenty-four hours later the Board of Public Works announced that city employees would do the work if the municipal treasury would provide the funds. A few businessmen tried, without success, to prevent compliance. The inspector also ordered the installation of cuspidors to cope with some of the accumulation of filth on floors that were customarily subjected to a flushing with water about once a week.[24]

The campaign technique had its limitations, for two years later, Brown again dealt with problems growing out of the unsanitary conditions of the farmers' market. A decision in the case of Jack Walters, a jobber, during April 1911 hindered constructive efforts. Walters's attorney pleaded that the Sanitary Food Law was unreasonable and that standards set by it were impossible to attain; the jury acquitted the defendant. In July, Brown obtained warrants for the arrest of several men operating booths in the market, but when they promised to conform, he obligingly agreed to drop the charges.[25]

Later, in mid September, Squire Dan U. Burke, a Nashville justice, bound over twenty butchers to the criminal court on bonds of $250 each for failing to screen fresh meat. Assessing the action taken, Brown recalled that he had tried to improve the market since 1909. He added: "The requirements of the food inspection were put on the lowest point consistent with protection of public health, as I realized the city intended building a new market house as soon as possible, and hence I wanted to work a minimum of hardship on stall owners. The latter, however, failed to appreciate the situation and continued to sell their foods under insanitary conditions, also failing to comply with promises made to me."[26]

Perhaps the campaign was the best tactic available because of the magnitude of the problem, the small size of the department, and the difficulties in securing convictions when Brown did reluctantly take cases to court. Apparently the inspector remained convinced of this, for in 1912 he used the technique in Memphis, a city he had rarely visited between 1908 and 1911. Mr. Crump's Memphis had a reputable city health department, and Brown had relied heavily on the services of G. W. Agee (a prominent bacteriologist) and other local health officials there during preceding years when appropriations were lean. They had managed to secure several convictions.[27] In April, Brown and two of his assistants, Dr. L. J. Desha and Dr. John Frick, arrived in the river city. The press announced their arrival and warned of "sad times ahead for those whose records in the state lab are not clear." While the officials were in town, authorities there imposed fines on two dealers who had not screened the doors and windows of their shops. Brown, however, recommended a minimum penalty for C. M. Dinstuhl, owner of a candy store, who saturated his cherry chocolates with brandy.[28]

The relative success of the campaign technique merits attention, for it was a common procedure employed by state food and drug officials. It was not altogether unlike the prohibition raids used first at the state level and then by federal authorities, although the raid was secret whereas the campaign was often announced in advance by the press with the objective of obtaining compliance with the law rather than sensational convictions. Both the prohibition raid and the campaign had their faults, usually the failure to force conformity over a long period of time. The seven years that Brown served can be used to a limited extent in measuring the success of the campaign technique (see table).[29]

Year	Number of Samples Food	Percentage Adulterated	Number of Samples Drugs	Percentage Adulterated
1908	206	54.40	......	....
1909	261	42.53	343	71.14
1910	128	43.70	204	64.30
1911		Figures Not Available		
1912	220	45.00	367	56.10
1913	181	49.72	185	40.54
1914	213	39.80	156	61.50

The percentages for these years showed that food adulteration, with slight fluctuations, declined over the seven-year period. Drug samples generally improved in quality except in 1914, when the department devoted more time to narcotics than ever before. The decline in the adulteration of food may have been more significant than these figures indicate; by 1913 Brown reported to the governor that his inspectors searched for illegal goods only, giving little or no attention to those believed to be legitimate.[30]

Very little of a definite nature can be derived from these figures in trying to measure the success of the campaign technique. Generally, however, it led to short-term, clean-up efforts which had to be revitalized periodically by renewed campaigns and the constant vigilance of authorities. Those who violated the law out of ignorance were gradually enlightened and tried to conform. Balky merchants who opposed the law sometimes complied, at least outwardly, for fear of gaining undesirable publicity and losing customers. Flagrant offenders continued to violate the law if they could afford to lose customers or if they catered to a caliber of people who remained uninformed or unconcerned; seemingly, they had little to fear in the way of prosecutions and fines.

Convictions were difficult to obtain, and Brown was lenient toward offenders, often accepting their word that they would conform and allowing them to escape prosecution. Concerned principally with securing pure food and drugs for the state, not with inflicting severe punishment, he issued warnings first and brought charges later. Nonetheless, he prosecuted a number of cases that were dismissed at the whim of the presiding judge or the jury. Two important cases went against Brown. In the first case he took to court, a petit jury acquitted Joseph Ezell, a former president of the Retail Grocers and Merchants' Association, when he was charged with selling oleomargarine as butter. The Jack Walters case likewise ended in a dismissal when a jury responded to the defense attorney's argument that the Sanitary Food Law of 1909 was unreasonable.[31] These setbacks revealed to Brown that the judicial system was content with the warnings that he issued but was not necessarily willing to inflict punishment when these warnings went unheeded. Brown found it far easier, however, to prosecute Negroes and foreigners. Every successful conviction under the Sanitary Food Law of 1909 involved Negroes or individuals with foreign names. A total of eight Negroes paid fines, along with B. Haiman, Xavier Faucon, and Tom Velasco, all of Nashville, and John Canale of Memphis.[32] This may have reflected a racial bias of Brown's, or, more likely, of the judges' and juries'. In any event, it seems highly improbable that Negroes and foreigners were alone in violating the Sanitary Food Law.

The fines collected during any particular year between 1908 and 1912 probably never exceeded $260. The official reports contain totals for only two years, 1909 and 1912. In 1909, $260 was collected; in 1912, $195. The maximum fine meted out to any single dealer during these two years was $25; the minimum, $5.[33] Newspaper coverage of arrests and convictions tends to substantiate the conjecture that $260 was probably the largest sum collected in one year. Total fines in 1914 under the Anti-Narcotics Law, however, may have exceeded earlier figures slightly, for some $50 penalties were imposed on physicians who issued prescriptions illegally.

When these feeble amounts are compared to fines and convictions in the neighboring state of Kentucky during 1906 and 1907, when convictions seemed to be especially numerous, the difficulty of enforcing the Tennessee law becomes clear. Food experts in the Blue-Grass State secured a total of 268 convictions and had 153 cases pending at the time they issued a report. During this period, the Division of Food Control, headed by Robert M. Allen, working out of the Agricultural Experiment Station in Lexington, cooperated with Louisville health officials to obtain a pure milk supply. They secured eighty convictions of men who were charged with feeding distillery slop to cows and keeping dairy animals in filthy stables. Each offender received a fine of $100 and a jail sentence of fifty days, the latter suspended when the defendant promised to cease such practices. These eighty convictions alone netted $8,000, which was recycled back into the Division of Food Control to cover operating expenses.[34] In Tennessee, fines could be used only for publication costs.

What success Brown managed to achieve in bringing about conformity to the law could be attributed in large part to public health education. Efforts in this direction were rather constant throughout his service in Tennessee. He relied on lectures, bulletins, circular letters, and displays. In 1914 he issued weekly press releases which found their way into small-town newspapers. One of his more interesting ventures centered on an essay contest for school children. Cooperating with the superintendent of public instruction, Brown offered two medals, first and second prizes, for the best themes dealing with hygiene or public health. The subject for 1910 received the awesome title "The danger to health from the common housefly and how it might be avoided."[35]

On the lecture circuit, Brown remained active. In addition to periodic discussions with civic groups, he offered to deliver two lectures annually, free of charge, to each medical college in the state. The colleges took him at his word, and he found himself speaking in Knoxville, Chattanooga, and Nashville. Sometimes visual aids complemented the lectures. When employees of the department prepared an exhibit dealing with patent medicines and false weights and measures for the Fiftieth State Fair, it was also displayed at other large public gatherings.[36]

If money were available for printing, the department issued a bulletin each year; the bulletin of 1910 was typical. Using language that the layman could understand, the inspector dealt with different subjects affecting public health. This publication, released in July, included such topics as the dangers of canned products and patent medicines. Metallic caps and containers posed a serious threat because they were made of lead and zinc, elements capable of entering into combinations with the acid in such food products as peppersauce and vinegar. Brown sometimes demonstrated such reactions, before live audiences, by placing a nail in a canned product and allowing a coating to accumulate.[37]

In the same bulletin the inspector revealed his apprehension of drugs and patent medicines. Much of his early work centered on headache remedies. Distinguishing between eyestrain and that particular variety of pain "which has its origin only in the cold gray dawn of the morning after," he denounced those cures that were supposed to alleviate suffering no matter what the cause. Brown claimed that most of these products were derivatives of coal tar or opium and that when used in large amounts, they caused changes in blood composition, depression of the heart, and sometimes stupor, coma, or death. Habitual use could lead to addiction, as well as to death.[38]

Such publications as the bulletin of 1910 went to any state resident who requested them. The Pure Food and Drug Department, as a rule, dealt more closely with urbanites than with rural dwellers; but Tennessee remained an agrarian society during these years, and therefore the inspector tried to win the support of farmers. In 1910, Brown, a farmer himself, addressed the delegates to a state agricultural meeting in Nashville. In this speech he outlined the ways in which the Pure Food and Drug Law benefited them. Dairymen, he claimed, profited when illegal practices of competitors were halted; and efforts to keep bleached flour and mixtures of ground meat and cereal off the market increased the demand for high-quality sausage, hamburger, and flour. Fruit growers prospered from regulations preventing the sale of acetic acid as pure apple vinegar. Because sorghum was of considerable importance to farmers in Tennessee, Brown admitted his concern that adulterated molasses competed with high-grade products. In commenting on impure drugs, he said that the farmer had more at stake than other citizens because his livestock as well as his family were threatened.[39]

Although farmers were victimized by food and drug swindlers, some of them had no objections to duping their customers, as the following exchange illustrated:

DELEGATE: What about making cherry jelly out of blackberries?
BROWN: I have never heard of a man doing it. I would like to catch him though.
DELEGATE: I have it at my house.
BROWN: What do you add to it, a little hydrocyanic acid?
SAUNDERS: Leaves of the cherry tree.
BROWN: That is the same thing.
DELEGATE: It makes good cherry jelly, all right.
BROWN: Don't you sell it for cherry jelly where I am.[40]

Aware of the delight that some farmers took in marketing exotic goods and in duping agents of the department, the inspector included a recipe for the manufacture of imitation cider in Bulletin Number 3, and he commented that most of the product formerly sold in the state had been artificial. Alerting consumers, he listed the stomach-revolting ingredients, which included one hundred gallons of rain-water, six gallons of honey, five ounces of powdered alum, and two pounds of yeast. Brown recommended that this concoction ferment for at least fifteen days before the addition of eight ounces of bitter almonds and the same amount of cloves. After it had set for twenty-four hours, two or three gallons of good whiskey should be added.[41]

Public health education, although of merit, had its limitations. To enforce effectively the laws entrusted to him and to implement his policies, Brown found it imperative to increase the number of employees in his department. Every report he filed with the governor included renewed pleas for additional appropriations. At the end of one year as food and drug inspector, he asked for more funds to enable him to hire two assistant chemists on a full-time basis, a part-time chemist during busy months, a laboratory helper, and a stenographer. During 1909 he began to realize his dream for a full-fledged departmental staff. He hired an assistant chemist at a salary of $1,800, recently provided by the legislature. L. J. Desha of Cynthiana, Kentucky, accepted the position. Although he had no experience with the enforcement of food and drug laws, he had earned a doctorate in chemistry from Johns Hopkins University; he possessed a thorough background in his discipline; and he came highly recommended both personally and professionally. Less than a year later, Brown reported to the governor that his work had been "eminently satisfactory."[42]

Desha remained with the department until 8 September 1912, when he accepted a professorship in chemistry with the medical college of the University of Tennessee. He was replaced by C. L. Bliss, a graduate of Cornell University who had had many years of practical experience as a chemist. Previously he had been employed by the University of Michigan and had been involved with government service in the Philippines. Another chemist, W. F. Purrington, worked with Brown and Desha during 1909 on a temporary basis.[43]

In 1910, Brown again asked the governor for aid in securing additional appropriations. The most pressing need of his office at that time, he claimed, was a proper force of inspectors with scientific training, not political hacks. The next year he was able to hire two men as inspectors at a salary of $1,200 each.[44] Before the end of 1911, when the department was beset with political difficulties, it had grown to a four-man, full-time staff with some temporary paid help and several volunteers.

Although the actual number of paid employees remained inadequate to perform the responsibilities assigned to the department, volunteers helped to reduce the work load. In accordance with authorization extended by the Board of Health, Brown commissioned worthy citizens throughout the state as special agents to aid in enforcement of the Sanitary Food Law. Mrs. Max Bloomstein, Mrs. Porter McFerrin, and Mrs. W. L. Arnold, active members of the Nashville Housekeepers' Club, were the first appointees. Other agents included Blaine Dudley and his assistants, W. L. Lyon, E. F. Corbett, and W. P. Moody, all of whom were involved with market inspection in Nashville; Dr. and Mrs. S. S. Crockett of Nashville; P. L. Shute, J. N. Anderson, and Dr. B. G. Tucker, health officials of Davidson County; G. W. Agee of Memphis; and Dr. Ben H. Brown of Chattanooga.

TENNESSEE PURE FOOD AND DRUG DEPARTMENT AS IT DEVELOPED FROM 1909 TO 1911

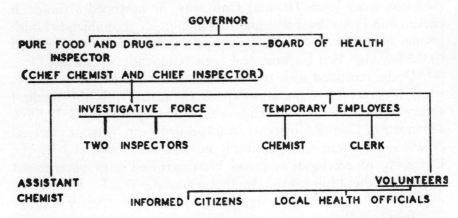

These special agents voluntarily inspected places where food was manufactured, stored, or sold and determined whether such locations were sanitary. City and county authorities performed these duties in addition to their regular obligations. Brown found this type of cooperation highly satisfactory, and he continued to appoint agents from Shelby and Davidson counties and from the cities of Nashville and Memphis. He originally adopted this policy after conferences with municipal officials who requested coordination of state and local health work.[45]

Brown devoted most of his time and energy to his official duties, but he also had strong loyalties to his profession. From 1908 to 1911, as he established a firm foundation for his department, he maintained his ties with professional organizations and earned a national reputation for himself as a food and drug official. In 1910, as a delegate of the National Association of Official Agricultural Chemists, he attended the Pharmacopoeial Convention in Washington, D.C., which was revising the United States *Pharmacopoeia*. The next year he presented a paper, "The Need of a Professional Code of Ethics among Chemists," to the American Chemical Society meeting in Indianapolis.[46]

The matter of professionalization and the image that chemists had of themselves received careful attention from Brown. In September 1909 he wrote to his friend Dr. Wiley: "It seems to me that the average commercial chemist comes nearer being a fool when the matter of compensation is concerned than any other man I know of. He does not seem to mind at all being placed on the plane of the shoe factory operative who does piece work and is perfectly willing to let the client set his fees so long as he is able to exist. It is very much to be desired that some body like the British Society of Public Analysts be organized in the United States." Wiley agreed that such a society might be desirable, provided that the agency itself could be financially independent and composed of men who would not issue false certificates.[47]

All of these professional concerns were subordinate to Brown's affiliation with the Association of State and National Food and Dairy Officials. From 1908 to 1911 he attended every annual convention. Although he had established connections with the association as early as 1904, it was not until 1909 that he became actively involved in the internal political struggles that plagued it. Most of the disputes centered on food standards and the use of preservatives. The problems surfaced in Theodore Roosevelt's administration, resulting in Dr. Wiley's fall from grace. Wiley himself dated his loss of favor from 1907, when the subject of using saccharin as a substitute for sugar arose. Wiley told the president that saccharin was a threat to health; Roosevelt answered angrily, "Anybody who says saccharin is injurious is an idiot"—his doctor gave it to him every day. After this incident, Roosevelt appointed the special Referee Board of Consulting Scientific Experts, who were in effect reviewing Wiley's work. Relations between the president and the chief chemist never improved.[48]

When the Association of State and National Food and Dairy Departments met at Mackinac Island in August 1908, Brown heard Edwin Fremont Ladd, food commissioner of North Dakota and president of the association, attack Secretary of Agriculture James Wilson for helping create the Referee Board. According to Ladd, the board represented the manufacturing interests. The entire organization joined the North Dakota delegate, going on record as regretting Wilson's stand and opposing the addition of any chemical preservative to food. Wiley, who attended the meeting, failed to defend the secretary as vigorously as he might have done, for he agreed with the substance of the attack. After this his position continued to deteriorate within the administration, and rumors circulated that he would be asked to resign.[49] Delegates to subsequent conventions of the association harbored the animosities of the pro-Wiley and anti-Wiley forces until the chief chemist resigned in 1912.

The convention at Denver in 1909 split over the benzoate-of-soda question. Secretary Wilson, determined to defend his views, headed the federal delegation but allowed Wiley to attend at government expense. The chief chemist, however, did not consider himself an official delegate. Nonetheless, he was busy behind the scenes, helping to organize a committee to report on benzoate of soda. He also operated through his friend Robert M. Allen to win the support of doubtful state delegations. Local reporters noted the existence of two distinct camps, warring for control of the convention. The Wilson faction managed to elect one of its own men as president, but the Wiley forces elected the vice-president, Lucius Polk Brown.[50]

The inspector from Tennessee had spoken against the use of chemical preservatives in food, as he explained later to the governor: "Believing that there was at least a doubt as to the healthfulness of such preservatives in foods; that they permitted the use of unsanitary methods of packing, and that such methods were opposed to the spirit of existing law in Tennessee, I was not in favor of admitting these materials to be used in foods."[51]

Brown had followed the Wiley philosophy—namely that all food additives posed potential dangers to human health—since his appointment in 1908. Through correspondence and personal contact at professional meetings, Brown and Wiley exchanged ideas, reviewed convention activities, evaluated laws, and discussed standards. Closely aligned professionally, the state inspector and the chief chemist developed a warm friendship—enough so that Brown could write to Mrs. Wiley that he would send her a dog, probably one of the Airedales he bred, if she could persuade her husband to agree. Brown added, "I did not dare say it to him, but I may say it to you, that his feeling with regard to dogs is the only blot that I have found on an otherwise perfect character." He indulged in a pun, revealing some of the frustrations of food and drug officials, when he suggested that Wiley did not like dogs because he had experienced so much hounding.[52]

The state inspector staunchly defended the views that he shared with Wiley in other conventions that followed the meeting in Denver. The organization remained fragmented when delegates gathered at New Orleans from 29 November to 2 December 1910. Again a dispute arose over the election of a president. Brown had the support of the Wiley faction. When the delegates deadlocked, six men—three from each faction—went into conference to try to come to an agreement. This resulted in a promise by the anti-Wiley people that if another man were chosen president, they would support Brown in 1911. Charles D. Woods of Maine, one of the men involved, gave the following account:

> I went to this candidate with two others and said to him, "I have betrayed you, you cannot be the President of this Association at this time, but it is agreed that you will be the President at the next convention"; and this man hesitated a moment and held out his hand and said, "It is all right," and this same man, when it came to the election of officers, made a nominating speech. . . . If you haven't read it, you should do so, as it shows the true character of the man. It shows that he can sacrifice all personal feeling for the good of the cause for which we stand. He accepted defeat that was given him at the hands of his friends and placed in nomination his rival.

With the Tennessee inspector willing to compromise, George L. Flanders was elected president; Brown, first vice-president.[53]

During the following year, Wiley's problems became more acute. The quarrel within the administration erupted openly in 1911, when Secretary Wilson charged that the chief chemist had acted irregularly in 1907 when he had employed Dr. Henry H. Rusby as pharmacognosist. In a cabinet meeting that took place while Wiley was out of town, Wilson called for his resignation. When the chemist learned of his plight, he released the details of his story to the *New York Times*. Many of his fellow citizens and his professional colleagues bombarded President Taft, Secretary Wilson, and congressmen with praise for him. The president, realizing the political inexpediency of dismissing Wiley, exonerated him in September.[54]

When the Association of State and National Food and Dairy Inspectors met in Duluth during August, the controversy over Wiley quickly became the dominant issue. Early indications were that the anti-Wiley forces were not going to honor the commitment to elect Brown as president, whereupon Woods reminded the convention of the earlier agreement, although two other men involved said they could not recall it. Nonetheless, Woods nominated Brown. The vote that followed was close, with 49½ votes for Dr. William P. Cutler of Missouri and 52½ for Brown. Robert M. Allen reported to Wiley that the likelihood of a tie had been so great that Brown cast a vote for himself because the Missouri commissioner would not forbid his delegation to vote. When the election was assured, Cutler moved that it be made unanimous.[55]

Brown's victory received immediate attention in Tennessee. The editor of the *Nashville Tennessean and American* called it "a merited honor" and one that Brown would bear with credit to himself and his state. He concluded: "Dr. Brown is the right man in the right place. His election was a Wiley victory, which means that poisoned foods and unwholesome concoctions will have no protection at his hands."[56]

By 1911, Brown had built a gradually expanding bureaucracy, made strides in educating the public, begun enforcing the laws in moderation, and risen to the highest office in a national organization composed of his peers. The inspector had little time to enjoy his professional triumphs or the praise heaped on him by admirers, however, for a struggle was shaping up that would require all the stamina he could muster to sustain himself. Since his appointment in 1908, the major political issue in the state had been prohibition. Clashes between opposing forces had resulted in a split in the Democratic party, in a state that had been solidly Democratic since Reconstruction. The result of the schism had been the election of a Republican governor in 1910. Meanwhile, businessmen in Nashville and Davidson County and the food and drug inspector had reached only a temporary truce at best. When Brown's second term expired in 1912 and the matter of reappointment had to be decided by Governor Ben. W. Hooper, those who opposed the inspector hoped to capitalize on the politics of the moment to rid themselves once and for all of the leading consumer advocate and health official in the state.

4—The Scientist
and State Politics, 1911-12

For almost four years, Brown kept his department free of the bitter partisan struggles brought on by prohibition. He was not as successful in this respect during the latter days of 1911 and the first three months of 1912. Those businessmen who opposed the work of the inspector attempted to convince Republican Governor Ben W. Hooper that Brown was a political liability, an incompetent, and an idealist. They misjudged the governor and failed to realize the importance of the public support that Brown had gained from 1908 to 1911. Still, the inspector's opponents created a furor over his reappointment in 1912 which, for a few weeks, put the future of the Pure Food and Drug Department in jeopardy.

As much as Brown the scientist would have liked to pursue his objectives in a political vacuum, he was a state employee; and no state employee, during the years he was in office, could have escaped completely the tensions that threatened to shatter the Democratic party. The impact of these serious divisions on the politics of the state can only be assessed when it is taken into consideration that this party had controlled state government since the termination of Reconstruction.[1] Once Middle and West Tennessee had been released from the home-grown radicalism of East Tennessee Republicans, the possibility seemed slight that this party would ever regain the power to dominate the state.

For a generation the Democratic party, which was composed of three distinct factions, settled into a routine of internal struggles, relatively untroubled by the possibility of the rebirth of a strong Republican party. The dominant faction, the old States' rights Democrats, was led by Isham G. Harris, the governor who took the state out of the Union in 1861. With their doctrine of secession in a shambles, this group came to be especially apprehensive of the ascendancy of federal power. The other older faction consisted of the small-farmer element headed, in turn, by Andrew Jackson, Andrew Johnson, and Robert Love Taylor. A third group, and the newest to enter the Democratic party, included the old Whigs from Middle and West Tennessee who had only with great reluctance turned secessionist. Actually this faction shared economic views with the East Tennessee Republicans. They preferred industrial and business development, whereas the other Democratic groups leaned almost exclusively toward agriculture.[2]

These factions, undisturbed by external political developments until the prohibition movement began to have serious influence, vied for control of the party and the state government. As early as 1877, temperance elements had secured passage of the Four-Mile Law, a loosely written piece of legislation which outlawed the retail sale of intoxicating beverages within four miles of any school outside an incorporated town. Almost unnoticed at the time of passage, this law became the instrument for drying up Tennessee.[3]

After advocates of temperance tried unsuccessfully to add a prohibition amendment to the state constitution, they organized a party in 1883, which gradually increased in size and influence. Over the years, temperance leaders secured amendments to the Four-Mile Law, until by 1907 they had seemingly dried up the rural areas and the small towns. The prohibition issue soon led to a schism in the state between rural and urban areas. City dwellers who had originally favored local option viewed the threat of complete prohibition as totally undesirable. A bill passed the legislature in 1907 providing for the extension of the Four-Mile Law to cities of 150,000 if they reincorporated after the proposal was enacted. Prohibitionist sentiment prevailed in Knoxville, one of the four largest cities, and citizens voted two to one for recharter. Meanwhile, Nashville, Memphis, Chattanooga, and Lafollette had not succumbed.[4]

Prohibition in the cities became a dominant issue when the crusade of the teetotalers interjected itself forcefully into Democratic politics in 1908. Former Senator Edward Ward Carmack, backed by prohibitionists, tried to win the Democratic nomination for governor from incumbent Malcolm R. Patterson of Memphis, who was favorable to local option but was an opponent of statewide prohibition. Although Patterson triumphed in the primary and subsequently returned to the governorship, state prohibitionists refused to accept his victory as a popular rejection of prohibition.

After Carmack's defeat, he became editor of the *Nashville Tennessean* and used his columns to crusade for prohibition and to lambast his political opponents. Unfortunately for Carmack, but most fortunately for the temperance spokesmen and teetotalers, the editor ridiculed Duncan B. Cooper, one of Patterson's chief supporters, a close friend, and an advisor. Cooper warned him that Nashville was too small to hold the both of them. On 8 November 1908, Cooper, accompanied by his son Robin, met Carmack by chance on Seventh Avenue, then known as Vine Street. Bullets began to fly, and when the smoke cleared, Carmack lay dead. Apparently he had fired the first shot, but a bullet from Robin's gun had killed him.[5]

Worth more to the prohibitionists dead than he had been alive, the late editor became a martyr. In January 1909 the General Assembly outlawed liquor in the state. Patterson vetoed the bill, but the legislature overrode him. After the Cooper-Carmack shooting, the governor's political stock continued to decline, but his pardoning of Duncan Cooper, who had been convicted of murdering Carmack, after the state supreme court upheld the trial court's verdict, spelled the political demise of Patterson and signaled a split in the Democratic party. Democrats who were inclined toward prohibition broke away from the Regular Democratic party. In the fall of 1910, Patterson withdrew from the gubernatorial primary, hoping to heal the wound precipitated by prohibition. He was too late to unite the party. The Independent Democrats joined with the eager Republicans to form the "Fusionist" movement and elected Ben W. Hooper, a Republican from Newport, over the aging Senator Robert Love Taylor, a holdover from the old small-farmer element and a recognized conciliator.[6] The election of Hooper marked the demise of the old three-faction

Democratic party. Prohibition had altered the state's dominant party and had brought about the election of the first Republican governor since 1880.

These were the political conditions under which Brown worked. With prohibition as the foremost consideration of state politicians, other issues received only superficial attention. Given the webs of kinship and political allegiance that existed in Middle Tennessee, almost everyone took a side. Brown, himself a relative of the Coopers, maintained a discreet silence on the liquor question.

Appointed in 1908 when the prohibition question rose to the highest echelon of state government, Brown remained relatively unaffected by the tumultuous political struggle until 1911. Nonetheless, politics remained an ever-present reality. The gentle reminder by Patterson that he expected support from his appointees, the suggestion that the inspector find a job for a certain young man named Fite, and a hint that hiring an elderly man, Tom Haynes, would be good politics, to say nothing of Brown's dependence on the legislature for operating funds—all kept him alerted to the true nature of his position. As loyal to his promise as a politician could be, Patterson left Brown free to run his department. He supported requests for additional appropriations, and he reappointed Brown on 23 November 1909, even though the first term did not expire until 15 January 1910.[7]

The inspector escaped the turnover of Patterson appointees when Hooper became governor because his second term did not expire until 15 January 1912. Nonetheless, Brown, a Regular Democrat, felt opposition building against him soon after Hooper was inaugurated. Not necessarily fostered by the governor, the opposition flourished in the political situation created by his success as a Republican candidate in the gubernatorial election of 1910. The editors of the *Nashville Tennessean and American* and the *Nashville Banner*, both progressive journalists with prohibitionist sentiments, had heretofore ardently supported the inspector's work, but what seemed to him a pointed editorial appeared in the *Tennessean and American* on 28 May 1911. Declaring that 250,000 children under one year of age died annually in the United States, a third of these from infected milk, the editor placed the blame on the authorities who "fail of their duty in bringing to account those who sell impure milk." He added: "Let us sharpen our wits and renew and increase our vigilance in giving proper care and providing pure and wholesome food for the babies."

Viewing the editorial as criticism of his work, even though in fact it may not have been, Brown responded almost immediately. In a letter, he argued that most officials were dedicated to public health. The real cause of infant mortality, according to the inspector, rested with public apathy and the meager appropriations of state legislatures. He placed the final blame on politicians: "Another and unfortunately potent element of opposition to these measures for the public good is 'peanut politics,' . . . and, while partisan politicians fight, the babies die." The editor accepted this explanation. At the end of June he insisted that liberal appropriations should be made for the enforcement of pure food and drug laws, and he praised the inspector for his accomplishments in spite of the limited funds at his disposal.[8]

The most serious opposition came, not from an occasional editorial, but from the organized merchants in the Nashville–Davidson County area. Disputes between the inspector and the businessmen which had arisen from 1908 to 1910 became public by the end of 1911. When Brown declared an all-out war on those who dealt in false weights and measures and instituted a grading system for establishments selling food, his enemies decided that the time was right to make their grievances known to the politicians.

In December 1911, Brown vigorously took up the work against false weights and measures. He swore out warrants for the arrest of twenty-five merchants. Most of the incriminating evidence had been gleaned by an undercover agent who bought an item and asked to weigh it on his personal scales, a practice that was distasteful to the merchants. Those who violated the law were summoned to appear before the pure food and drug inspector and explain their positions. Most of them presumably did not know the difference between a "wet" and "dry" measure. Some of the men blamed "country people" for selling them illegal products. The editor of the *Tennessean and American* chimed in that at last the time had come when the consumer was going to have a square deal.[9]

Although the merchants who were charged with violating the common law against false weights and measures and with mislabeling their products promised to cooperate in the future, the Retail Grocers and Merchants' Association agreed to meet at their hall in the Bruce Building on 7 December 1911 for the purpose of deciding how to cope with this new problem. M. T. Mallon, president of the organization, claimed that Brown was after the wrong men. Blaming farmers, Mallon charged that they always insisted that their measures be used in transactions with merchants. Mallon said that the businessmen had no intention of opposing the new ruling, although a few hotheads had suggested making a test case. After the meeting, Mallon notified the local newspapers that his group had endorsed Brown and had agreed to assist him in every way.[10]

If the businessmen were not disturbed enough already, Brown ended the year with another surprise. He established a grading system of "excellent, good, fair, poor, or bad" for all places selling food. A certificate bearing the grade had to be placed on permanent display in all food-handling establishments. This system had been used in Maine, Indiana, and Kansas, but no other southern state except Louisiana made widespread use of it. Although it was intended to be a positive innovation, Tennessee restaurant operators and grocers considered it to be yet another method of harassment.[11]

The adoption of grading, as well as the crusade against false weights and measures, immediately preceded the drive to oust Brown from office. While publicly promising to support these measures, members of the Retail Grocers and Merchants' Association secretly plotted to block his reappointment. Fully aware that Brown's term was about to expire, they increased their criticism of him. The citizens around Nashville and in other areas of the state began taking their positions on the matter of reappointment in December 1911. The pro-Brown group included local women's organizations, farmers, and professional people. The opposition enlisted the members of the local trade association. Between the two camps stood Lucius Polk Brown, "the visionary and dreamer and incompetent" or the "Dr. Wiley of Tennessee." With the end of his second term approaching, he was caught in a cross fire of insults, accusations, and endorsements.

Businessmen cast Brown as a liability to Hooper. Enemies charged that the inspector had never given a Republican a job, although D. J. Frazier, a subordinate inspector, had once campaigned for the post of representative from Cumberland County on the

Republican ticket. A Nashville newspaper, in defense of the inspector, claimed that several of his appointees had voted for Hooper. In any event, Brown had not voted for Hooper in 1910. He gave his support to him, however, when he ran in 1912, although he was under the general impression that it was too bad that the man was a Republican.[12]

Alert to the political turmoil in the state, Brown had anticipated the controversy surrounding his reappointment. Almost immediately after his election to the presidency of the Association of State and National Food and Dairy Inspectors, he began mobilizing his supporters. His old colleague, Dr. Wiley, an experienced warrior in political feuds, drafted a letter to Governor Hooper in September, praising the inspector and suggesting that he be reappointed. He gave it to Brown unsealed and told him to use it as he thought best; Brown mailed it to the governor.[13]

In late December, when the fight was on, Brown once again took up the matter with Wiley. He suggested that the chief chemist might speak to the governor on his behalf when Hooper visited Washington. He revealed his personal opinion of the state executive to Wiley: "Governor Hooper has made us a good Governor so far, has stood for the right as nearly as possible, has not been swayed by machine motives in his appointments or actions, and I think that I can work effectively for the public interests with his administration." When the governor went to the national capital during January, Wiley called on him at the Willard Hotel. He found Hooper absent, but he left a message that he had been there to pay his respects. Later, a friend of Wiley's revealed to him Hooper's remarks on learning of his visit: "I know what Dr. Wiley wants to see me about. It is about the appointment of a food commissioner."[14]

Hooper was aware of Brown's national reputation and the possibility of adverse criticism of his administration if the veteran inspector were not reappointed. He also understood the commercial-agrarian schism in the state. At times, hostility between the agrarian and commercial interests almost superseded the issue of reappointment as each group tried to shift the blame for false weights and measures. Neither farmers nor storekeepers were as blameless as they would have liked to appear, and farmers might never have concerned themselves with the reappointment issue had they not come under attack from Brown's enemies.[15]

As the merchants became more vocal in their opposition to reappointment, other supporters of Brown entered the fight. Two women's organizations of Middle Tennessee were among the first to express favorable opinions of the inspector. In December, members of the home section of the Middle Tennessee Farmers' Association adopted resolutions commending him. The Centennial Club of Nashville, a group of homemakers numbering approximately five hundred, endorsed Brown and asked for his reappointment. According to an editorial in the *Tennessean and American*, the women spoke "in unmistakable terms."[16]

Although Brown's supporters included nonfarming groups, the agrarian-commercial struggle persisted. One man wrote to a Nashville newspaper, commenting that he would probably have to pay to get his letter in print. Addressing Brown, the writer said that he was obligated to express his appreciation because work "against the universal dishonesty of the mercantile world" greatly benefited his class.[17] F. O. Beerman, who did not identify himself as a farmer or as a merchant, succinctly expressed the opinion of the agrarians. While congratulating the inspector for his efforts to protect the consumers, especially those of the "ignorant and poorer classes," Beerman declared that it was nonsense for the public to blame the farmers for short weights. He further asserted that merchants took care of their interests first, without thought for the customer. "The endeavor to push this proposition on the farmer is all buncombe," said Beerman, "for any child 7 years old knows that in each case the merchant takes care of himself."[18]

Brown agreed that his purpose was to protect the small consumer, adding:

> In the work done up to date, it is manifest that it would be an injustice to any one man or set of men to publish their names, for the reason that everybody has been doing it. It is a universal custom, and might bring undeserved odium upon a well-meaning man. But parties in this state are now warned what to expect, and hereafter not only prosecutions will be brought, but publication will be made. Moreover, in

all cases which have heretofore come before us in which guilty intent seems to exist, publication will be made.[19]

Thomas P. Calhoun, a farmer of Davidson County, also replied to charges that the farmers were to blame for incorrect measures. Calhoun claimed that if a farmer refused to use the buyer's measure, he would be told very quickly "to drive on with his load." Then he scoffed at the idea of a man carrying his scales to weigh his products or of a retailer accepting another measure than his own. To clinch his arguments, he added, "As farmers, we have not complained against Dr. Brown, so we are not the hit dog, for we have not howled." He suggested that if farmers had ever imposed "on the poor retail grocerymen, let them report us to Dr. Brown and have him make it hot for us." Calhoun reaffirmed his support for the inspector and the law when it was administered equally to businessmen and farmers.[20]

On 4 January 1912 the strategy of the businessmen took on a new dimension when they carried the case against Brown to Governor Hooper. The delegation, comprising forty to fifty men, met the governor behind locked doors because they did not want the public to know who was against the inspector. One man declared that they fought Brown, not for personal reasons, but because of "his incompetency." He said that the official was "impractical and visionary" and ignorant of the weights and measures used by businessmen. Brown, some contended, employed mere "boys" who might ruin a man's reputation. Other merchants claimed that the grading system adopted by Brown in late 1911 discriminated against the small businessmen who could not afford to stock or furnish their stores as lavishly as wealthier merchants. The meat dealers complained about the ruling that their products be kept under glass, adding that if meat were kept in a glass case, more clerks would be needed to remove it. The dissident merchants further alleged that the pure food and drug inspector had directed a whirlwind campaign to have himself reappointed. Governor Hooper thanked all of them for their opinions and informed them that he had also been approached by Brown's supporters.[21]

After the businessmen met with the governor, representatives of the medical and teaching professions added their voices to those of farmers and housewives in support of Brown. The Nashville Academy of Medicine and the Davidson County Medical Society unanimously endorsed him and sent the resolutions to Hooper. These groups usually avoided active support of candidates seeking political offices, but because of the concern of the medical experts with public health, they made an exception.[22]

Another endorsement came from W. R. Webb, headmaster of the Webb School at Bell Buckle. After calling attention to the changes in food preparation from homes to factories, he announced his belief that the general public, not just the citizens of Nashville, were interested in the appointment of a pure food and drug inspector. He admitted his ignorance of the validity of the charges made by the grocers, but still considered the state blessed to have a man of the caliber of Brown. He remarked on the similarity between this struggle and the one that involved Dr. Harvey W. Wiley. He pointed out that Wiley's influence and prestige had been enhanced. He added that he thought the same would be true in Brown's case. Webb assumed that Hooper would not make the mistake of removing an efficient officer, especially in view of his interest in progressive programs involving prisons, education, and agriculture. In conclusion, the educator challenged the Nashville merchants to invite customers to inspect their places of business.[23]

Not a man to remain silent when under attack, Brown, in a letter to Hooper, answered the charges of the Retail Grocers and Merchants' Association. His office, he insisted, performed necessary functions. Moreover, he had requested the cooperation of the merchants, but many of them had failed to respond. He firmly denied that he had discriminated against anyone. His publication of names was authorized under the Pure Food and Drug Law of 1907. In answer to an assertion made by some businessmen that he "never molested soft drink stands," the inspector said that in 1911 he issued 48 orders for changes to the owners of such stands in Nashville, 496 throughout the state. This particular criticism may have been designed to persuade the governor that Brown allowed the operators to sell liquor illegally, a practice not unusual to soft-drink stands. The inspector himself disliked these businesses and thought anyone a fool who would pay five cents for a bottle of carbonated water. Brown also defended his legal right to establish a grading system.[24]

The conflict between the agrarian and urban interests continued in the midst of the reappointment controversy. The editor of the *Tennessean and American* said that if grocers cheated farmers, then a definite need existed for uniformity in weights and measures. John Coode, a grocer, defended his associates by declaring that they were not villains or "short weight artists." The unpleasant situation, he said, could have been avoided if the legislators had made sufficient appropriations for the operation of the Pure Food and Drug Department. He innocently added that adequate funds would have allowed Brown to consult with experienced grocerymen. M. T. Mallon again hoisted the banner of the businessmen by blaming farmers for providing them with unsatisfactory goods. He staunchly denounced the rural people who caused the grocers to be falsely accused.[25]

The term of the pure food and drug inspector expired on 15 January 1912. Hooper had failed to act on the matter of reappointment by this date. The governor responded with a great deal of political acumen by asking Brown to remain in office until a successor could be named. This was an indication that he intended to appoint a new man. Leaving Brown in the position, however, gave cause for optimism among his supporters. By avoiding a formal commitment, Hooper maintained a balance between the two groups and gave tempers time to cool.[26]

On 1 March 1912, a month and a half after the second term expired, Hooper reappointed the veteran inspector. In his formal announcement, the governor said that he had been elected on a law-enforcement platform, and Brown had distinguished himself by an honest effort to enforce the law. He further praised his fairness and his attempt to keep his department from becoming a political arena. The governor subtly hinted that perhaps Brown had not been as diplomatic and considerate as he might have been. Nevertheless, he attributed these difficulties to the establishment of a new department.[27] Reappointment of Brown by the Republican governor was an important landmark for the department, raising it above partisanship.

If the press reflected general sentiments, then the governor's decision was a wise one. In East Tennessee the *Knoxville Sentinel* and the *Knoxville Daily Journal and Tribune* carried stories of the fight. The editor of the former wrote that opposition to reappointment would be undesirable publicity for businessmen speaking out against the inspector. The editor commented that Brown appeared to be conscientiously enforcing the laws. The inspector enjoyed favorable coverage by the *Chattanooga Daily Times* when he urged, during his first year in office, that the mayor and councilmen appoint a municipal pure food and drug inspector for that city. The *Nashville Banner* and the *Nashville Tennessean* supported Brown from the time of his initial appointment by Governor Patterson in 1908. Because of insufficient funds, the inspector had left much of his work in Memphis to the city health officials; but the *Commercial-Appeal* praised Hooper when he announced the reappointment.[28]

Undoubtedly, the governor gave considerable thought to the matter before he revealed his decision. Although very active and highly vocal, the Nashville Retail Grocers and Merchants' Association constituted only a minority of voters in one well-defined area of the state. They simply realized the possibilities for exploiting a rare political situation to rid themselves of pure food and drug enforcement by preventing the reappointment of a conscientious official. They were numerically weak, and their arguments lacked validity. They also left themselves open to criticism from both city and country dwellers, presented an undesirable image, and seemed unwilling to do everything possible to safeguard the consumers. Their confrontation with farmers proved unwise in a predominantly rural state where many citizens still believed sincerely in the arcadian myth.

The weakness of the Nashville–Davidson County merchants' position was complicated by the fact that they were not completely united among themselves and that they certainly did not speak for all businessmen in the state. Brown received a letter from C. T. Cheek & Sons of Nashville, informing him that they had ordered the employees in all their stores to sell by weight and asking him to force their competitors to do likewise. These businessmen aded: "It will be quite hard for us to continue selling by weight unless you force our competitors who are selling by measure to give the correct weight." They suggested that Brown instruct his inspectors to test the weights of products where grocers sold by measure. Another group, the Board of Directors of the Southern Poultry and Egg Shippers' Association, adopted a resolution praising Brown which was forwarded to the governor.[29] Support from such areas as these revealed the minority position of the merchants who opposed the inspector.

As much as some businessmen would have liked to pit a realistic professional politician against an idealistic scientist, Hooper and Brown could not be cast in these roles. Even if Hooper had been swayed by the rumors that Brown was a political liability because he was a Regular Democrat who never gave a Republican a job, he was in no position to take a partisan stance. No viable two-party system existed in Tennessee at that time, and Hooper would never have occupied the executive mansion had it not been for the intrusion of prohibition into state politics, resulting in a schism within the Democratic party. He was not a machine politician but more of a gentlemanly reformer put into office by a fusion effort. With the exception of his endorsement of prohibition, Hooper was similar to his Democratic predecessor. Both were inclined toward moderate reform. Both were also politicians—although Patterson was more of a professional than Hooper—and hence opportunists; and probably the truth of the matter was that except on the prohibition question, both men occupied virtually the same position on the political spectrum.

Whereas Patterson at one time had enjoyed the advantages of a strong Democratic machine, Hooper had only the backing of wayward Democrats and a weak Republican party, united temporarily by the common bond of prohibition. To be reelected in 1912 he needed the support of many of the very groups whose representatives urged him to reappoint Brown. The number of scientists in Tennessee was small. Therefore, the inspector could not rely exclusively on his professional colleagues to exert enough influence to secure his reappointment. There were, however, enough professional people in the state to make their voices heard. The governor could hardly have ignored the endorsements of the medical societies or the arguments put forth by the old educator "Sawney" Webb. An Independent Democrat, Webb had served as chairman of a conference in 1905 which agreed to endorse any measure that would abolish saloons by extending the Four-Mile Law or by giving wards in "wet" cities the right to prohibit liquor sales.[30] When professionals joined with home-makers, farmers, and the state press in their support of Brown, his reappointment was almost inevitable; for these were the types of people who had originally installed Hooper in the governorship. The anguish of this one episode, magnified many times by other small controversies and added to the major issues, inspired Hooper to recall in later years that his administration was "unquestionably the most turbulent political period in the history of Tennessee, not excepting even the era of Reconstruction."[31]

As the storm over the reappointment subsided, friends of Brown's began a campaign to have him named chief chemist of the United States Department of Agriculture, the post formerly held by Dr. Wiley. On 16 March 1912 the *Washington Times* carried a story in which Brown was mentioned as a possible successor. The reporter also gave the details of his association with the national pure food and drug movement and of his administration in Tennessee. Several prominent citizens joined the effort to win the post for Brown. Chancellor Kirkland of Vanderbilt University; P. P. Claxton, head of the National Education Bureau; Hilary Howse, mayor of Nashville; and the members of the Vanderbilt chapter of Beta Theta Pi sent letters and telegrams to President William Howard Taft. Luke Lea and others from the Tennessee congressional delegation also endorsed Brown.[32]

In the meantime, Brown remained silent. He was in Hillsville, Virginia, attending the funeral of his brother-in-law Judge Thornton Massie, who had been murdered while presiding at the trial of the Allen brothers, members of a moonshining clan. When the inspector returned to Nashville, he expressed appreciation for the efforts of those who sought his appointment as chief chemist. He indicated, however, that he had no desire to hold that office. Although he promised to write to Taft and explain his position, some Tennesseans, among them a local traveling men's organization and members of the Nashville press, continued to endorse him. Brown never took the action seriously, but the newspapers kept the issue before the public until December 1912, when Dr. Carl Alsberg was appointed.[33]

After the excitement of reappointment subsided and the drive to secure a federal position for Brown had waned, the veteran inspector returned to the pursuit of his old objectives. Enlarging the department, educating the public, and campaigning against businessmen who sold illegal products occupied most of his time. He also maintained his association with the national pure food and drug movement. In March he attended a meeting of the National Civic Federation Committee in Washington, D.C., where prominent officials discussed food and drug control in the United States. In July, as its president, he addressed the Association of American Dairy, Food and Drug Officials. In that speech, he assessed the progress made in stemming the adulteration of food and drugs. Admitting that court actions had gone against enforcement officials at all governmental levels, he maintained a spirit of optimism: "The future of food and drugs control work in the United States appears bright. Despite the great amount of work still to be done, the public is so vitally interested in the subject, and public enlightenment thereupon has been so much advanced that public support should be more general in [the] future and more freely rendered."[34] Brown understood well the importance of public support. It had kept him in office in 1912.

Reappointment did not offer Brown tranquility. In addition to making numerous inspections, writing reports, and delivering speeches, he found himself in court as plaintiff and defendant. In November 1912 he was on the defensive. The Homeopathic Specific Medicine Company sought an injunction to stop his interference with the sale of its products.[35] The case was eventually dismissed when the company agreed to comply with existing laws.

The year 1912 marked the zenith of Brown's career as state pure food and drug inspector. From meager beginnings in 1908, Brown had secured considerable support for his position from the average citizens, from newspapermen, and even from some businessmen. The reappointment controversy revealed the attitudes of the population in the state shortly after the turn of the century. Representatives of the teaching and medical professions especially were interested in reform. Many of the farmers and businessmen shared an animosity for each other that was out of proportion to their concern for correcting the ills of society. Surprisingly enough, Brown maintained his composure as a public servant and his concern for the health of the people in the midst of a battle between forces that were not so dedicated to social welfare. He had proved himself and his department in 1912. From 1913 to 1915 it became clear that instead of destroying or weakening the department, the businessmen had succeeded only in enhancing its reputation. Even with partisan struggles still under way, the governor and the legislators seemed determined to raise the department above their bickering. The Republicans and the divided Democrats joined together in a nonpartisan spirit during the special legislative session of 1913 to double appropriations for pure food and drug enforcement. Although the inspector continued to serve in Tennessee for another three years, this period would prove anticlimactic when compared with the first two terms.

5—From Southern State to Northern City: The Scientist in Professional Transition

Between 1913 and 1915 Brown continued to enforce the Pure Food and Drug Act of 1907 and related laws in much the same manner as in the previous years. Appropriations increased substantially as the General Assembly provided for employment of additional personnel and more effective investigation. Opposition that had plagued the department from its beginnings subsided tremendously, as did the general political turmoil in Tennessee, evidenced by the reunification of the Democrats to elect Tom C. Rye governor in 1914. Doubts and suspicions on the part of lawmakers and citizens gave way to a concern for improving the Pure Food and Drug Department, and Hooper's reappointment of Brown to a fourth term in 1914 went virtually unnoticed. Unfortunately for Tennessee, Brown resigned a year later to assume a post in New York City. Before he left the state, however, he had established a viable department and publicly accepted procedures of operation.

The Fifty-eighth General Assembly, which convened in 1913, gave Brown an opportunity to present his plans for the Pure Food and Drug Department when the Assembly created a special commission to investigate the department's needs. Although both his duties and his staff had increased sufficiently to justify his use of the title of commissioner, he continued to have visions of an even-larger enforcement agency. Asking for no increase in his own salary, he requested funds to hire another chemist, three additional inspectors, a laboratory assistant, and a porter.[1]

During its first four years of existence, the Pure Food and Drug Department had grown noticeably. By 1913, Brown directed the work of two full-time inspectors, an assistant chemist, a few temporary employees, and several volunteers, and he supervised the enforcement of three major laws. The future of the department during the remainder of Brown's service was settled by the work of the General Assembly. The controversy of 1912 had strengthened his position with the governor, and Hooper recommended to a joint session of the legislature that the Pure Food and Drug Department be "increased in scope and usefulness." In his message, Hooper lauded earlier accomplishments: "It is but just to state that no department of the State government has struggled harder and against greater odds to enforce the beneficial laws within its jurisdiction than this department." He also suggested that the lawmakers read the report outlining the department's financial needs.[2]

Political squabbling continued to haunt the General Assembly, and this dampened the commissioner's hopes for substantial increases in appropriations. Bills designed to ensure Regular Democratic control of election machinery set off controversies that resulted in boycotts of meetings by Independents to prevent the formation of a quorum. Brown wrote to Dr. Wiley that political maneuvering prevented the passage of food and drug legislation although public sentiment favored progressive action. So little was accomplished during the regular term that Governor Hooper called the legislators into a special session, which was scheduled for 8 September.[3]

By September the failure of the legislature to act responsibly threatened the effective enforcement of existing food and drug laws and the Sanitary Hotel Act of 1911, which had been assigned to the Pure Food and Drug Department. This measure required hotel operators to install lights, fire exits, and extinguishers; to maintain sanitary rooms and clean kitchens; and to provide individual towels, sheets, and toilets. The Tennessee Travelers, an organization of salesmen who had lobbied for the bill, exerted pressure to promote adequate funding of the department. As a result of their efforts, the reputation of the work already accomplished, and memories of the reappointment controversy, which had been fraught with arguments based on the lack of funds, the legislature voted $25,860 annually for the maintenance of the department over the next two years. In contrast, the appropriations for 1911 and 1912 had totaled only $11,200 per annum.[4]

With the additional money the commissioner added a few more employees than he had anticipated in earlier years, but extra responsibilities accompanied larger appropriations. In one of his "Weekly Chats with Consumers," Brown wistfully traced the development of his department from its frail infancy to its sprawling adolescence, noting: "The Legislature of 1913 was liberal to the Department in giving four additional field inspectors, and an office force of two persons, but they were almost as liberal with duties."[5]

TENNESSEE PURE FOOD AND DRUG DEPARTMENT AS IT DEVELOPED FROM 1912 TO 1915

GOVERNOR

PURE FOOD AND DRUG — — — — — — — — — — — — — — — —BOARD OF HEALTH
COMMISSIONER

INVESTIGATIVE FORCE	OFFICE STAFF	TEMPORARY EMPLOYEES
SIX INSPECTORS	CHIEF CLERK	DETECTIVE
	PORTER	CLERK

CHEMISTS   VOLUNTEERS

TWO ASSISTANTS   LOCAL HEALTH OFFICIALS
                                                                     CITY POLICE

New legislation affecting the department in 1913 included a series of bills to prevent false weights and measures, an act placing all employees except the commissioner under civil-service regulations, and an antinarcotics law. Since his first term, Brown had requested action on standard weights and measures. In January 1913, S. W. Stratton of the Bureau of Standards in Washington, D.C., advised Governor Hooper that the Eighth Annual Conference on Weights and Measures would be held from 14 to 17 May. He requested that the governor appoint a delegate. Before the meeting took place, Hooper informed Stratton that Tennessee had no statute dealing with standard weights and measures and therefore was in no position to be represented effectively. The governor referred the matter to Brown. Legislators came to view this situation with concern, and that same year, Frank E. West of Knoxville and other representatives secured the passage of three bills. The first made statutory the common-law prohibition of the sale of short weights and measures; the second created a state department of weights and measures; and the third established standard weights and measures for Tennessee.[6]

The governor appointed Brown to the position of superintendent of weights and measures. After a year the commissioner reported that 30 percent of the 2,939 weights and measures inspected were inaccurate, and he estimated that 83 percent of the linear and 75 percent of the liquid measures were no better. To illustrate the unfair burden on consumers, Brown suggested that if 550,000 families in the state spent as much as $180 annually for groceries, a total of $99 million, they lost at least $4,195,000 through false weights alone.[7]

In addition to enacting weights and measures laws, the legislators placed employees of the Pure Food and Drug Department under civil-service regulations. This seemingly removed the positions from the realm of political patronage. All applicants for inspection work had to be tested. The examinations dealt with practical questions related to the laws, spelling, arithmetic, penmanship, report writing, and commercial geography as well as training, experience, and fitness. A new employee remained on probation for six months. If he proved unsatisfactory at the end of the trial period, he was informed in writing of the reasons for the termination of his services. The power of the governor to appoint the commissioner, however, could undermine civil-service requirements. Some animosity arose because George Draper, a pharmacist from Gainsboro who had been recommended by Governor Hooper, received a temporary appointment without first having to undergo the examination. Apparently the job was a favor granted by Hooper to his friend W. W. Draper, the father of George Draper. The younger Draper eventually underwent the perfunctory test and thus retained his position.[8]

As commissioner, Brown assumed responsibility for the conduct of several lesser officials. Attempting to keep his department in smooth running order, he vacillated between benevolent paternalism and harsh discipline. On 17 March 1915 he made the following entry in his diary: "Had to can Von Sholly—being steadily insubordinate and lack of teamwork. He seems to be utterly unfit for work of this class by temperament and training—I understand his people are well-to-do, which explains a good deal of it." Von Sholly must have been inept, for Brown usually displayed a forgiving nature. When Lewis Titcomb, an inspector, reported expenses that seemed to be above normal, Brown chastised him severely. He vowed to himself to "make a man of the boy yet," and he soon reported that he had "Titcomb straightened."[9]

The old educational and enforcement objectives were still pursued, but Brown delegated much of the responsibility for them to his trusted subordinates. Public health education, which had been fostered by the department since 1908, lost some of its personal touch between 1913 and 1915, when it was redirected from the old lectures before small audiences toward techniques that commanded the attention of large groups. The efforts during 1913 and 1914 were limited almost solely to an exhibit dealing with adulterated food and drugs. It appeared in Knoxville at the National Conservation Exposition. Later, the commissioner, with the governor's approval, allowed the Russell Sage Foundation to take it to Atlanta. The American Interchurch College returned the display to Nashville, and later it showed up in Memphis sponsored by the Young Men's Christian Association.[10]

Widespread newspaper coverage became more common than lectures. In 1914, Brown issued frequent press releases, describing such matters as the dangers of patent medicines, the importance of public cooperation, and the development of the department since 1908. They appeared in the columns of weeklies throughout the state.[11] The new appeal to mass audiences marked a maturation of the department from its early days when the commissioner had taken to the stump in major cities and minor burgs across Tennessee just to secure enough support from taxpayers to perpetuate the office that he occupied. Brown believed that he no longer needed to sell the idea of pure food and drug control, and therefore he simply kept the attention of the public focused on the work of the department.

During his last years in the state, Brown moved to enforce the Sanitary Hotel Law of 1911 more vigorously than before. Instituting the old campaign technique, he announced in early October 1913 that within a ten-day period, the six inspectors would tour the state, checking hotels for violations. In January 1914 he closed the McKenzie Hotel of Nashville because of dangerous and unsanitary conditions. Although the law had been in effect long enough for hotelmen to comply, Brown and D. J. Frazier, an inspector, agreed to review the property again after repairs had been made. Two members of the Tennessee Travelers complained when the order was issued because the lodging was conveniently located near the railway station. Brown replied, "The boys secured the law and are demanding its enforcement, so they must take their medicine." In March, Brown shut down another hotel, the Arlington in Johnson City. During 1914 the officials inspected 435 facilities, some more than once, issued 355 notices for corrections, and eventually awarded 247 certificates.[12]

Routine work occupied the staff, but the commissioner devoted the remainder of his service in the state to enforcement of the new Anti-Narcotics Act, which went into effect on 1 January 1914. His concern with addiction grew out of his efforts to force correct labeling of patent medicines and out of his contacts with drug users in the pursuit of his duties. The legislature had charged the state food and drug inspector with the responsibility for enforcement of the Anti-Narcotics Act, but he shared the task of drawing up guidelines with the secretary of the Board of Health. The law itself limited the dispensing of cocaine and opium compounds to registered physicians, dentists, and veterinary surgeons in the course of professional practice only; to registered pharmacists filling legitimate prescriptions; and to wholesale dealers who made distributions to the appropriate people. All purchases and sales had to be recorded.[13]

The striking feature of the law centered on the provision that allowed addicts who registered as such to acquire a supply of narcotics. The legislators had two reasons for including this section. First, they believed that the state could not afford to build and maintain hospitals for treating users. Therefore, to salve their consciences, they decided to minimize suffering by allowing habitués to procure drugs. Second, they hoped to prevent an illegal traffic in such contraband.[14]

Not all physicians had the understanding of and the concern for humanity that were possessed by legislators, the commissioner, and the secretary of the Board of Health. During March 1914 a detective employed by the Pure Food and Drug Department arrested two doctors, W. B. Hager and H. B. Hyde, and charged them with selling and distributing prohibited drugs. He had gone to the offices of the accused and had obtained prescriptions for an alleged friend. Issuing such prescriptions violated the law. In the criminal court of Davidson County, the doctors based their defense on the invalidity of the legislation and on the manner in which evidence had been procured. Judge A. B. Neil upheld the law and found the defendants guilty. Dr. Hyde appealed the case to the state supreme court. In December, Justice Samuel C. Williams, representing the eastern division, delivered the decision, which supported the verdict of the lower court. Dr. Hager, meanwhile, continued to trouble the commissioner. The doctor had an irritable disposition and had accosted Brown on numerous occasions. Once he swore out a warrant, charging Brown with assault. The court imposed a fine on the commissioner "to insure peace in the future between them." At the time, Chancellor J. B. Newman, who presided, remarked illogically that he believed Brown innocent.[15]

In the spring of 1914 the commissioner carried the fight against narcotics from Nashville to Memphis. Several physicians were indicted in West Tennessee for selling dope. While in the city, Brown read before the state medical society a paper entitled "The Drug Habit in Tennessee from the Viewpoint of an Enforcing Official." He estimated in 1914 that between 5,000 and 10,000 addicts could be found in the state, with more women involved than men. He said that the first goal in enforcing the law was to stop illegal sales by physicians.[16]

After the law had been in effect twelve months, 2,370 people—blacks and whites, men and women of all ages—had registered as addicts. Brown indicated that this figure probably did not include even half of the drug users in the state. Of those who obtained permits for prescriptions, 784 were male; 1,586, female. Women addicts outnumbered men by more than two to one, with the greatest preponderance ranging in age from 25 to 44; men, 35 to 64. Not over 10 percent of those registered were Negroes, although that race composed about one-fourth of the total population. The commissioner explained that the average Negro tended to avoid contacts with public officials.[17]

Brown believed that real and imaginary illnesses led to the use of drugs. Women between the ages of 25 and 55 represented 63.5 percent of all female addicts. Problems related to childbearing and menopause probably caused them to seek relief through drugs. For men also, he surmised, suffering from various illnesses—including venereal diseases, which "accounted for no inconsiderable proportion of the trouble"—contributed to addiction. He found also that addicts were more common to West Tennessee than East Tennessee. The former had a ratio of 1 addict to 928 people; the latter, 1 to 1,359. Brown credited climate for this development. East Tennessee, he said, had "a salubrious and rather bracing climate," whereas marshy West Tennessee, lying between the Mississippi and Tennessee rivers, fostered malaria, which caused considerable suffering among the residents of that section.[18]

The commissioner's stand on narcotic control was tolerant for the times in which he lived. The program launched in Tennessee resembled the approach taken by Dr. Charles E. Terry in Jacksonville, Florida. As city health officer, Terry established a drug clinic so that habitual users could receive free narcotic prescriptions. This limited the excessive profits of unscrupulous pharmacists; it also removed the influence of the medical profession through its power of prescription. Terry and Brown both believed that physicians were largely responsible for causing addiction. Neither was optimistic about private sanitaria, which were associated in the public mind with moral turpitude and the spread of vice and crime.[19]

Even as the controversy over the treatment of addicts raged, Brown voiced his findings on addiction in Tennessee, as well as his personal opinions, at the 1914 convention of the American Public Health Association; and he appealed for careful consideration of the issues. If state institutions for drug users were not available, he favored the policy adopted in Tennessee, where addicts received drugs legally. When he concluded his speech at the meeting in Jacksonville, Florida, he pleaded "for an intelligent and scientific study" of drug addiction. Commenting on the attitude of physicians toward the subject, he said: "It is so new, and the mental position of the large majority of the medical profession toward it has been of such a nature, that it has not had from alienists and from men specializing in allied fields the attention to which its importance entitles it." In his final statement he reminded the association: "The drug addict is a sick man both physically and mentally, and should be studied and treated as a sick man and not as one always wilfully delinquent."[20]

Enforcement of the Anti-Narcotics Law presented Brown with a new challenge, and court cases kept his last days as commissioner filled with excitement. As both plaintiff and defendant, he ended his service on the note of sensationalism that had characterized many days of his administration. Occasionally, Brown encountered manufacturers of adulterated products who possessed a zealous belief in their powers. Such was the case of John S. Akin, the general manager of Vital Remedies Company of Houston, Texas, who became involved in a suit during January 1915. Brown believed that Akin was "more honest than the average patent-medicine man," but that he had hypnotized himself into a faith in the medicine. "Vitalitas," the product in question, was composed of a mixture of disintegrated clay and shale—which had no apparent healing value. The case against the company was eventually dismissed when Akin agreed to label his product correctly. The suit, in which Brown was the defendant, grew out of a quarrel with W. D. Walker, who had been arrested for violations of the weights and measures statutes. The irate Walker had Brown prosecuted for carrying a deadly weapon. The absurd case never went to a jury. Under the laws of Tennessee, any officer with police powers, while engaged in official duties, had the legal right to carry a pistol.[21]

The petty suits, political squabbles, and problems arising from the creation of a new department had taken their toll on Brown's health. He found the summer climate of Tennessee depressing, and his frequent bouts with gastritis were undoubtedly brought on in part by the strains of the job. In 1915 he was forty-eight years old, personally ambitious, and had a wife and four children to support. The position he held offered very few, if any, opportunities for advancement. His salary had never risen above the $2,500 that he had received from the first year of his service, although new responsibilities continued to increase. He was state superintendent of weights and measures, state hotel inspector, and pure food and drug commissioner; and from his vantage point, it seemed that he was being drained of all his energy and talent without adequate financial compensation. Although he had never requested a raise for himself, Brown had every right to expect one. Furthermore, the verbal commitment of politicians to enforcement of statewide prohibition threatened to subvert the real purpose for which his department had been created.[22]

Tennesseans had embarked upon the noble experiment of prohibition, and state officials could not afford politically to show a lack of concern in dealing with enforcement of the liquor laws. Since 1909, when the General Assembly had attempted to banish alcoholic beverages from the state with the so-called bone-dry law, additional legislation had been passed to ensure the "teetotalism" of state residents. The Democrats, outwardly at least, accepted the situation and launched an effort to reunite the party, which had split in 1909 over the liquor issue. In 1914 they nominated Tom C. Rye of Paris, a party regular who had been attorney general in the Thirteenth Judicial District. Acclaimed as a candidate of the masses, especially the rural people, he called for enforcement of the liquor laws and disclaimed any connection with the liquor interests or city bosses. Rye won the election for governor in November, defeating Republican incumbent Ben W. Hooper. Democrats also gained control of the General Assembly.[23]

In a message to the legislature on 18 January 1915, Rye pleaded for the passage of measures to halt the practices of illicit liquor dealers. The lawmakers responded with three new laws, two of which involved the Pure Food and Drug Department. The first of these dealt with soft-drink stands, which were denied the right to sell any beverage containing more than one-half of one percent alcohol by total weight. Responsibility for enforcement fell on the pure food and drug commissioner. A second law affecting the department denied druggists the right to dispense intoxicants without a valid prescription.[24]

Because of the strengthening of the liquor laws, Brown found his department charged with ferreting out alcoholic beverages in drugstores and at soft-drink stands, with an implied responsibility of raiding dives, alleys, barns, stables, private clubs, and homes. A Regular Democrat and a dedicated food and drug advocate who on special occasions sometimes celebrated with a drink, the commissioner viewed these new obligations with disdain. The demands placed on his department ran counter to his personal and professional beliefs. He mustered enough interest, however, to receive praise from the East Nashville Women's Christian Temperance Union for his work in suppressing "the unlawful dope habit and the illegal selling of whiskey" in their city.[25] By 1915, conditions in Tennessee caused Brown to look favorably on opportunities elsewhere. Such was his state of mind when the New York City Department of Health announced a competitive examination to select a new director of the Bureau of Food and Drugs.

As undesirable as New York City might have seemed for a product of rural Tennessee, the position there held certain attractions for Brown. Professionally, it offered more possibilities for advancement and financial compensation than the job in the South. Brown, as well as most other health officials in the country, regarded the New York City Department of Health as a model organization. Furthermore, the position of a bureau chief carried a salary of $5,000, twice that of pure food and drug inspector in Tennessee. Also, the New York office appeared to offer more security. Brown's retention of his post in Tennessee rested with the discretion of the governor. Although the employees in the department were hired on the basis of competitive civil-service examinations, the position of chief inspector depended on political appointment. For all of these reasons, Brown applied for the job in New York and prepared to undergo the written examination.[26]

The commissioner's service to the state rapidly came to an end. On 24 April 1915, Robert W. Belcher, secretary of the Municipal Civil Service Commission of New York City, notified Brown that he was among twelve men who possessed the experience and had passed the written examination for the position of director in the Bureau of Food and Drugs. Belcher also summoned him for an oral examination in New York during early May. Brown was suffering from influenza and doubted whether he would be well enough to appear. Nevertheless, he recovered sufficiently to make the trip, and he left for the North on 30 April. The examination consisted of hypothetical questions related to the enforcement of pure food and drug laws.[27]

When the Tennessean applied for the position in New York City, he had reason to be optimistic. Along with considerable ability as an administrator and scientist, he had influential friends and relatives there. Even before the great trek of rural black and white southerners to the northern cities occurred during the early decades of the twentieth century, a few hardy souls had drifted northward in search of economic and professional opportunities. One such individual was William M. Polk, a son of Confederate General Leonidas Polk's and a cousin of Brown's. A prominent physician, he occupied a seat on the Medical Advisory Board of the New York City Department of Health during 1915. It had been Polk who had encouraged Brown's brother Ewell to practice medicine there. More than any other family member, cousin Frank L. Polk, son of the physician, wielded considerable influence in city politics. As corporation counsel and personal friend of Mayor John Purroy Mitchel, he was in a position to help Brown. Along with family support, Brown had an acquaintance who served on the Civil Service Commission. A Miss Upshaw, the daughter of A. B. Upshaw of Columbia and Nashville and the granddaughter of Houston Thomas of Maury County, took particular interest in his application. Frank Polk described her as "one of the right hand men" on the commission.[28]

On 3 May, Brown learned that he had scored 90.60 percent, surpassing Marion B. McMillan, who was director of the Bureau of Food and Drugs, and the highly respected Robert M. Allen, head of the Food and Drug Division at the Kentucky Agricultural Experiment Station. Shortly thereafter Brown was offered the job. When the time actually came to make a decision on his future, he found himself in a dilemma. The New York position seemed to hold enormous professional opportunities. Nonetheless, some risks were involved. As a family man, he realized the problems inherent in uprooting his children from their rural home and plopping them down in such a metropolis as New York City. The family enjoyed a comfortable life on their twenty-five-acre farm at Franklin, a commuter village near Nashville that provided its residents with the best of country and city living. Brown, too, enjoyed the attachment to the soil, and he found relaxation in growing vegetables, raising animals, and breeding Airedales. Therefore, instead of severing all ties with Tennessee, he decided to ask Dr. R. E. Fort, president of the State Board of Health, for a leave of absence, beginning 21 June, to give him time to make a permanent decision.[29]

As soon as the announcement was made that Brown had been offered the New York position, he was swamped with congratulatory telegrams and letters from ordinary citizens, club women, professional people, and politicians throughout his native state. Tennesseans received the news of his impending departure with mixed emotions. Although most of his acquaintances were pleased with his success, they were concerned about finding a qualified replacement. One communication that Brown must have found especially gratifying, given his concern for addicts, came from a drug user who expressed his appreciation for the efforts that Brown had made on his behalf and for others like him.[30]

Having been granted the leave of absence, Brown left his family in Tennessee and departed for New York toward the end of June. On his way north he stopped in Washington, D.C., to discuss the directorship with his friends at the United States Department of Agriculture. Willard D. Bigelow, head of the food division, seemed to think well of the opportunity; and Dr. Carl Alsberg, chief chemist, looked even more enthusiastically on the offer. Brown, however, wrote to his wife that he hoped "not to be stampeded."[31]

When Brown arrived in Gotham he took up residence at the Chemists' Club, 52 East Forty-first Street, and occasionally spent time at the home of his brother. At the Department of Health he was well received by his colleagues and found the conditions "very fine." He established a satisfactory working relationship with Dr. S. S. Goldwater, the health commissioner. The assistant director of the bureau, a Swede named Ole Salthe, who was a veteran of eleven years, pleased Brown very much. The new director concluded that he had "made a hit" with those of his men whom he had met. He wistfully commented, "There are 155 of them—so I haven't met them all, by any means—I hope I shall do so some day." He soon made distinctions between his old position and the new one. "Of course I am not the 'big man' as I was in Tennessee," Brown said, "but inasmuch as my Bureau is one of the most important in the Department, and such of the public as are interested in the matter are watching this somewhat unique experiment with some interest, I fancy people won't forget our existence."[32]

By the end of June, Brown had decided to give up the position in Tennessee. He informed Governor Rye of his plans while the state executive was in New York on business. Brown, who kept his wife posted on new developments, wrote to her: "I broke the 'sad news' to him. I think the matter looked much less serious to him at this distance. Don't say anything about it until he lets the matter out."[33]

Meanwhile, Governor Rye was faced with the responsibility of finding a suitable replacement to serve out the term, which was due to expire on 15 January 1916. Several state residents imagined themselves to be qualified for the position, and they bombarded Rye with applications and numerous recommendations, usually written by personal friends and family. Under serious consideration for the post were George Draper, a registered pharmacist from Gainsboro who had been employed in the department for a while; W. H. Hollingshead of Nashville, a graduate of Vanderbilt University and an employee of the Pure Food and Drug Department, who was recommended by Brown; George C. Childress from Knoxville, also a graduate pharmacist trained at Vanderbilt; and J. E. Justice of Clarksville, a pharmacist who established headquarters at the Hotel Hermitage in Nashville to conduct his campaign for the job. Justice, too, had been graduated from Vanderbilt and had taught there for six years before entering the retail drug business.[34]

The leading contender for the vacant position was Harry L. Eskew, something of a dark horse, who came to Tennessee in 1903 as the southern representative of Sharpe and Dohme, a pharmaceutical company of Baltimore. A native of Ohio, he had received his education in the public schools there and later had earned a degree in pharmacy from the University of Cincinnati. In addition to being a member of the Travelers Protective Association, Tennessee Travelers, and

United Commercial Travelers, he was a prominent Mason and belonged to the Knights of Pythias. The members of the Nashville Manufacturers' Association, the Commercial Club of Nashville, and the Tennessee Pharmaceutical Association rallied to his support.[35]

Traveling men of Nashville and other interested parties gathered on Sunday, 11 July 1915, at the Tulane Hotel and boosted his campaign. Those present appointed a special committee to notify Governor Rye of their endorsement. Some confusion existed at the rally because of a misunderstanding as to the purpose of the summons by J. R. Bass and H. P. Fritz, presidents respectively of the Tennessee division and the Nashville post of the Travelers Protective Association. Fritz, contending that he had nothing against Eskew, stated that participants had the power only to consider the advisability of making recommendations. He later wrote to the governor, lamenting the endorsement of Eskew by the "drummers." Referring to him as "an eleventh-hour candidate," Fritz further asserted that Eskew was merely a man who was being endorsed by close friends and was not a competent chemist. He urged the appointment of someone who possessed the virtues of former Commissioner Brown. One of the traveling men, in his enthusiasm, forwarded a ridiculous statement to Rye, declaring that if the traveling men's candidate were appointed, "the Knights of the Grip" would be eternally grateful and from that time forward would be tied to Rye with "strong golden cords of sincere gratitude and appreciation."[36]

The "Firing Line," a section of the Sunday edition of the *Nashville Tennessean and American* devoted to the activities of the "drummers," contained an explanation of their interest in the appointment, along with more praise for Eskew. According to R. J. Cowan, former grand counsellor of the United Commercial Travelers, the traveling men's candidate was particularly well suited for the post because of his many years of experience on the road, his education as a chemist, and the fact that he was of the "very highest type of manhood." Cowan claimed that the travelers shared a particular concern because of their success in securing new laws and an increase in appropriations for the Pure Food and Drug Department. The United Commercial Travelers, the Travelers Protective Association, the Tennessee Travelers, and the Nashville City Salesman's Association represented strong pressure groups in the state. Collectively they had helped to obtain passage of the Sanitary Hotel Law of 1911 and an allocation of more than $25,000 for the department in 1913.[37]

Tennesseans in 1915 took the duties of the pure food and drug commissioner seriously, and many were concerned with finding a new one. An editorial in the *Tennessean and American* outlined the difficulties involved. According to this statement, published shortly before Governor Rye announced his choice, the position demanded a man of high integrity who was an expert chemist possessing administrative ability. The appointee, furthermore, would not find it necessary to do groundwork, for a suitable foundation had been established by the first commissioner.[38]

Governor Rye, apparently reacting to the pressure of the "drummers," announced the appointment of Harry L. Eskew, not a "chemist of established reputation and ability," as prescribed by law, on Saturday, 24 July 1915, at 1:00 P.M. He expressed his pleasure in making the choice and claimed that he had never had better authority for appointing a man to office than in this instance. Thirty minutes later, Eskew, wasting no time, appeared before Chancellor J. B. Newman and was sworn into office. Brown, in New York, viewed the selection of Eskew as "a politician's appointment." The governor, he thought, had made his decision "with reference alone to the enforcement of the liquor laws." The former commissioner added: "He could have had all he wanted in Hollingshead."[39]

In spite of Rye's selection of a man who was not qualified for the job under law and his failure to be influenced by the recommendation of the first inspector, Brown could reflect on his accomplishments in Tennessee with some satisfaction. Appointed to the newly created position of state pure food and drug inspector in 1908, he was assigned the tremendous task of creating an enforcement agency. He soon formulated objectives that called for development of a full-fledged department that would be involved with public health education as well as law enforcement. At the same time he pursued his own professional interests. After more than seven years he had realized virtually all of his early goals.

The one-man agency became a well-established department within four years. When it was tested by the issue of reappointment in 1912, it sustained itself and emerged stronger than ever before. The relative success achieved by Brown in his efforts to educate the public and to enforce the laws fairly helped the department through the crisis of 1912. While the commissioner himself was never quite satisfied with the size of his staff, he had succeeded in building a department that received favorable recognition from the people it served and from the politicians who controlled its fate. Nurtured by Brown from its infancy, the department survived his resignation but floundered under the direction of a new man who was not of the caliber of the first inspector.

The pure food and drug work in Tennessee during the Progressive era would have been of little consequence, in all likelihood, had it not been for the character and ability of the man who directed it. Living in a rural southern state that had limited financial resources and was less than five decades removed from the trauma of the Civil War and Reconstruction, Tennesseans of that period were very fortunate to have the combination of scientific expertise and public spiritedness to be found in Brown. His reputation was not limited to his own state. The high esteem in which he was held by his professional cohorts throughout the United States led them to elect him to the presidency of the Association of State and National Food and Dairy Inspectors in 1911. When he applied for the directorship in New York City, he put himself in competition with many of the country's foremost authorities, and he surpassed them all.

The arresting feature of Brown's position in Tennessee was the amount of freedom that he, as a scientist, possessed in formulating policy. Virtually unrestrained except by the possibility of not being reappointed after the expiration of each two-year term if he became a political liability, he continued to expand his department and to take on additional responsibilities that improved the stature of his department and increased his power. The political situation in the state allowed him to create a surprisingly large bureaucracy, considering that he served little more than seven years. No viable two-party system had developed, and the split in the Democratic party that accompanied prohibition left politics in flux. In the absence of a dominant bloc of highly professionalized politicians seeking to expand their own sphere of influence and jealously eyeing newcomers in the government, Brown enjoyed a great deal of flexibility.

When the commissioner resigned and accepted the directorship in the North, he was about to enter a wholly different political environment. The New York City Department of Health was well established; the hierarchy of authority was fixed; and the big-city professionals resented the presence of scientific reformers in jobs that could be used for political patronage.

6—The Scientist as a Northern Bureaucrat, 1915-17

With the move to New York, Brown loosened his ties with Tennessee and entered the uncertain environment of the nation's greatest metropolis. Because of financial limitations, the preponderance of his work in the South had been in the urban centers. The rural people, however, constituting the majority of the population, produced most of what they ate; in New York City, consumers, with the exception of a few suburbanites who had backyard gardens, depended exclusively on middlemen for their food supply. As director of the Bureau of Food and Drugs, Brown addressed himself to controlling the quality of raw products entering the city, those being processed, and the finished items being sold in the marketplaces. His experience in the rural South with its emerging cities could hardly have prepared him, psychologically, professionally, or politically, for the situation he faced.

The population of New York numbered more than twice that of the entire state of Tennessee, and its composition differed drastically. Tennessee possessed a population of 2,184,789 when the census was taken in 1910. Whites accounted for 1,711,432; Negroes, 473,088; Indians, 216; Chinese, 43; and Japanese, 8; and the "all-other" category took in 1 Hindu and 1 Korean. The overwhelming majority, 2,166,182, of the total residents were native born; only 18,607 were of foreign birth. On the other hand, New York City had a total population of 4,766,883. Of this number only 19.3 percent were native white and of native parentage. Native whites of foreign or mixed parentage constituted 38.2 percent of the total, and foreign-born whites accounted for 40.4 percent. Negroes represented only 1.9 percent. Therefore, 78.6 percent of the total population of New York City consisted of foreign-born whites or second-generation immigrants.[1]

The South, including Tennessee, had remained relatively free from the influx of the "new" immigrants that began in the 1880s. New York City, however, served as a port of entry for millions. A large percentage of these uprooted masses filtered into the core areas on the Lower East Side, found dwellings and jobs, and settled down to a subhuman existence until fate intervened to carry them to a heavenly reckoning. Others managed eventually to make a better life for themselves beyond the worst tenement districts.

The presence of these hundreds of thousands of aliens helped to make New York different from Brown's native state. Their numbers, their relative helplessness upon arrival, and their quest for a better life made them not only pawns of Tammany's great political machine but also problems for the Department of Health. No public official could remain unexposed to the influence of the Democratic organization for long. Brown, fortunate in this respect, moved to New York when Tammany was out of power. The mayoral election of 1917 would shatter the fragile dreams of many reformers, but for two years the director of the Bureau of Food and Drugs gave all his attention to the demands of his new job.

To acquaint himself with his responsibilities as director, Brown ventured forth into the slums with some of his men. He was both fascinated and horrified by what he observed. After one foray, he wrote:

> I went yesterday with some of my men into the congested district—you ought to have seen it! In the Ghetto crowds gathered in a second when we stopped—and push-cart dealers with exposed foods took to their heels when we were a block off. In Mott Street (Chinatown) I saw stuff I didn't know existed—dried oysters—dried "sea-ears" (something like a mussel)—and the like. In Little Italy and the Ghetto we saw them selling new and strange foods I never heard of—such as

squash-leaves and stems—and the squash-flowers seemed to be placed to one side as a special tid-bit.[2]

Despite the efforts to adjust himself to his new environment, Brown found it difficult to commit himself to these exotic surroundings and the strange hoards of people. Even after he had resigned from his position in Tennessee, he harbored misgivings about remaining in New York. In mid August he wrote to his wife that he had heard through the departmental grapevine that Commissioner S. S. Goldwater thought that he would make the best director there. In the same letter he revealed his doubts, resulting perhaps from nothing more serious than a bout with homesickness:

> But even with this and apparently success in hand, I am of late seriously wondering whether it will be worthwhile. There is no doubt that it is a hard place to live, and to bring up children in—and it is *not* American. The work is the most interesting I ever tried, and there are a lot of fine people here, but there are also a lot of the other kind. We shall certainly feel very much like fishes out of water for a while, and possibly we shall be longing for the country even though we get a place in the suburbs. . . . What do you think of my throwing it up and coming back home to make out the best we can for a while?[3]

Ambition had the upper hand with Brown, and toward the end of the letter, which was filled with misgivings, he outlined opportunities for advancement. At that time, rumors circulated that Frank Polk might run for mayor in 1917. Brown pointed out that his cousin seemed "to be universally popular and trusted." He then changed the subject from Polk to himself. If Goldwater should resign, the director noted, that did not necessarily mean that he would be replaced by a physician. Continuing, he said:

> Indeed, the position would appear to call more for good business management than for profound knowledge of medical matters, and when a little of both is combined, the success is reached that Goldwater is universally acknowledged to have met with. But it also opens the possibility of a man who has reached success as a manager, within the Department

itself, getting to be either Deputy Commissioner or Commissioner—so you see there are possibilities in this line that I did not calculate on when coming here![4]

Whatever doubts Brown had about the future he laid to rest. He continued to search for a family dwelling in his off hours, and on the job, he attempted to familiarize himself with the work of the bureau. By 20 September his probation as a new employee had ended, and with a sigh of relief, he boasted that "now only misconduct, inefficiency, or resignation, can pry me loose from this job." Reflecting on the trial period, he observed that it seemed "ridiculously easy" and that "the City of New York has not had very much efficiency in this position heretofore."[5]

With his job status now somewhat secure, Brown settled into a routine at the Bureau of Food and Drugs. He was not "the big man" that he had been in Tennessee, but according to the director, there was "almost as much to be done" as when he had become state pure food and drug inspector. Moreover, the Department of Health was a powerful organization with hundreds of employees under the supervision of scientific experts.

The New York City Department of Health during the Progressive period traced its origins from the establishment of the Board of Health there in 1866. The state legislature, responding to the recommendations of a citizens' committee, passed a law that reorganized health administration in the port city. In effect the legislature divided the state into two sanitary districts: the first being the Metropolitan Sanitary District, which comprised the counties of New York, Kings, Westchester, and Richmond and the towns of Newton, Flushing, and Jamaica, located in the county of Queens; the second being the remainder of New York State. Lawmakers placed the administration of the Metropolitan Sanitary District in the hands of a board of health, which was then made up of a president, the commissioner of health, the commissioner of police, and the health officer of the port, along with a few auxiliary officials. Health administration for the remainder of New York State lagged behind the metropolitan area until the 1880s, when the lawmakers created a state board of health.[6]

The Metropolitan Board of Health, as an administrative unit, changed very little for the next three decades; the scope of its work, however, broadened, and the number of employees increased. From an initial concern that was almost exclusively oriented toward dealing with epidemics of cholera, smallpox, typhoid, and diphtheria, the Board of Health came to have an interest in preventive medicine and laboratory methods. As a department, Health took on even more importance after the creation of Greater New York City. In 1898, officials spent a considerable amount of time taking over the health administration of the towns and villages that had recently been incorporated.[7]

Under the city charter of 1898 the Department of Health occupied a unique position in government administration. Not only was it exempt from practically all the health laws applying to the remainder of the state, but also its board acted as a legislature, which has been described as a "headless fourth branch" of city government. Under powers that were delegated by the state legislature and the city charter and were upheld by the courts, the board passed ordinances, which were embodied in the city's Sanitary Code, on all matters pertaining to public health. Therefore, the board represented an obvious exception to the time-honored tradition of prohibiting the delegation of legislative powers to administrative agencies.[8]

When Brown went to New York, the Board of Health still consisted of three members: the commissioner of health, the commissioner of police, and the health authority of the port. Two of these members, therefore, occupied their seats as appointees of the mayor. The third, a federal official, was somewhat removed from city politics. Because of the manner in which two-thirds of the members came to be a part of the Board of Health, that agency could be used rather forcefully in political matters if a mayor or particular party organization had the desire to do so. In any event, the efficiency of the Department of Health, in large part, depended on the judiciousness of the prevailing political party.

From the standpoint of general organization and departmental efficiency, the establishment of eight distinct bureaus between 1910 and 1914 seemed to be an improvement. They included: General

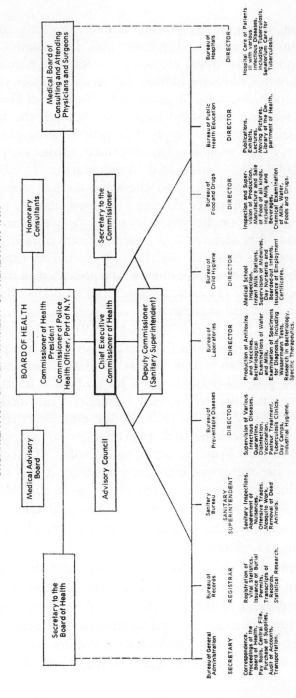

ORGANIZATION OF DEPARTMENT OF HEALTH IN 1915.

From New York City, Board of Health, Annual Report, 1915.

BOARD OF HEALTH
Commissioner of Health
President
Commissioner of Police
Health Officer, Port of N.Y.

Medical Board of Consulting and Attending Physicians and Surgeons

Honorary Consultants

Medical Advisory Board

Secretary to the Board of Health

Secretary to the Commissioner

Chief Executive Commissioner of Health

Deputy Commissioner (Sanitary Superintendent)

Advisory Council

Bureau of General Administration
SECRETARY
Correspondence, Proceedings of the Board of Health, Central File, Pay Rolls, Purchase of Supplies, Audit of Accounts, Transportation.

Bureau of Records
REGISTRAR
Registration of Vital Statistics, Issuance of Burial Permits, Transcripts of Records, Statistical Research.

Sanitary Bureau
SANITARY SUPERINTENDENT
Sanitary Inspections, Abatement of Nuisances, Offensive Trades, Mosquito Work, Removal of Dead Animals.

Bureau of Preventable Diseases
DIRECTOR
Supervision of Various Infectious Diseases, Quarantine, Disinfection, Vaccination, Pasteur Treatment, Tuberculosis Clinics, Day Camps, Industrial Hygiene.

Bureau of Laboratories
DIRECTOR
Production of Antitoxins and Vaccines, Bacteriological Examinations of Water and Milk, Examination of Specimens for Diagnosis, Including Wassermann Tests, Research in Bacteriology, Specific Therapeutics.

Bureau of Child Hygiene
DIRECTOR
Medical School Inspection, Infant Milk Stations, Supervision of Midwives, Day Nurseries and Boarded-out Infants, Issuance of Employment Certificates.

Bureau of Food and Drugs
DIRECTOR
Inspection and Supervision of Production, Manufacture and Sale of Food of all kinds, including Milk and Beverages, Chemical Examination of Milk, Water, Foods and Drugs.

Bureau of Public Health Education
DIRECTOR
Publications, Exhibits, Lectures, Moving Pictures, Library of the Department of Health.

Bureau of Hospitals
DIRECTOR
Hospital Care of Patients ill with various Infectious Diseases, including Tuberculosis, Sanatorium Care for Tuberculosis.

87

Administration, Records, Sanitation, Child Hygiene, Infectious Diseases, Food and Drugs, Hospitals, and Laboratories. During 1914, Commissioner Goldwater created one additional bureau, Public Health Education. Goldwater himself noted three major objections to the bureau plan. First, he observed that directors of the bureaus were too far removed from field inspectors. Second, the individual employee failed to grasp or apply the general principles of the department, and the monotonous, repetitive nature of the work inhibited mental and professional development. Third, various bureaus sent out representatives to the same districts and often to the same houses, which wasted time and annoyed citizens. Goldwater questioned whether these disadvantages could be overcome or if the bureau plan should be replaced by a system of local or district administration. In order to resolve the matter, he created an experimental health district, headed by a single chief who represented all the bureaus engaged in field work. The commissioner indicated that this experiment showed a great deal of promise.[9]

The political nature of the Board of Health combined with the commissioner's misgivings about the bureau plan to make a precarious situation for such bureaucrats as Brown. Ironically, he thought that he had escaped political troubles when he boarded a train for New York, believing that the civil-service regulations provided a great protective umbrella. When he realized, for example, that his pay would be docked if he went back to Tennessee to arrange for his family's move to New York, he wrote to his wife: "Of course in a huge organism like this government, administered as it is on strictly civil service lines, rules are necessary, and this is only one of the rules, so you must not think it unreasonable—it is quite the contrary."[10] If his opinion altered during his first two years in New York, he had little time to reflect on the change.

Large sections of the Sanitary Code dealt with food and drug standards. The code, however, outlined neither the specific responsibilities of the director of the Bureau of Food and Drugs nor those of other directors of bureaus in the Department of Health. Although these positions, the results of administrative shuffles, had civil-service sanction, they were not included in the Sanitary Code. The responsibilities of the director of the Bureau of Food and Drugs, according to a flow chart contained in the *Annual Report* for 1915, were to inspect and supervise the production, manufacture, and sale of all types of food and to examine chemically milk, water, food, and drugs. Commissioner Goldwater had also assigned the laboratories to Brown.

The new director, his duties broad and hazy, tended to define his responsibilities in much the same manner as he had during his tenure as state food and drug commissioner. In Tennessee he had concerned himself with four major objectives: increasing the size and power of his department, educating the public, enforcing the laws, and building a national reputation for himself. Although major differences existed between the Tennessee position and the New York situation, there were enough similarities to permit him to pursue his old programs by modifying them to fit new contingencies. In Tennessee, Brown had created a new department and operated on meager budgets; in New York he inherited a ready-made bureau within a mature department of the city government. The Department of Health had 3,059 employees in 1915, not including executive and advisory personnel, and a budget of $3,322,426.09.[11]

The origins of the Bureau of Food and Drugs within the Department of Health stemmed from the 1880s, when the officials in New York State as well as those in the largest city took an interest in the deleterious substances contained in food and adopted regulatory measures. The state legislature passed a pure food law in 1881. City health officials during the same decade made some efforts to control the milk supply there. When Ernest J. Lederle, acting chemist, injected milk from diseased cows into guinea pigs, they died. According to Charles F. Bolduan, director of the Bureau of Public Health Education, writing in 1916: "It is safe to say that this occurrence strongly determined Doctor Lederle's subsequent great interest and activity in the supervision of the milk supply. So far as the Board of Health was concerned, we find it constantly taking a keen interest in the milk supply and backing up the efforts of its administrative officers."[12]

For many years the supervision of the municipal food supply had been handled by the Sanitary Bureau. In 1912, however, Lederle, during his second term as commissioner of health, transferred the work to the newly created Bureau of Food and Drugs. It then assumed the functions of the old divisions of food and drug inspection, city milk inspection, and sanitary inspection. This change eliminated duplication of services. Under the former arrangement, a milk inspector, a food inspector, and a sanitary inspector might visit the same premises on a given day.[13]

With the centralization of the inspection force and the assignment of laboratories to the Bureau of Food and Drugs, the number of employees came to 188 in 1915. Not awed by the size of his force, Brown reacted to it as a bureaucrat seeking to sustain his private stronghold. According to him, the bureau had a shortage of inspectors. In 1916 he lamented that there were only 32 men assigned to milk control, whereas there should have been 140 or more. He also complained, with justification, that only 3 inspectors made up the drug division. Though the director had hopes of enlarging his staff, they came to naught. Official reports indicated that his bureau made virtually no additions during the period that he served.[14]

BUREAU OF FOOD AND DRUGS, 1915

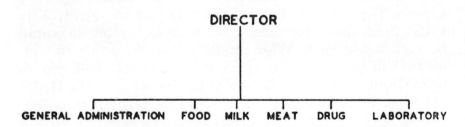

Since the bureau was already established and was employing almost 200 people, Brown decided that it was absolutely necessary that he become acquainted with them. His own success, in a sense, depended on the character of his employees and the rapport that he could establish with them. Soon after he arrived in the city, he made a habit of going on inspection tours with his men. By August he observed: "I seem to be getting at my force of food-inspectors, whose morale was in bad shape as a result of [the] previous Director's mistakes and incompetence." Social events provided him with additional opportunities to meet his employees. On 31 July 1915 the Food Inspectors' Association sponsored its first annual family outing and picnic at Morningside Park. All such former gatherings had been "stag." Brown attended and met most of the 175 inspectors. Later, on 5 February 1916, the food inspectors held a banquet in the Gothic Room at Murray's, 228 West Forty-second Street.[15]

Brown's interest in getting acquainted with his inspectors was stimulated, in part, by his well-grounded suspicion that some of them were accepting bribes from unethical food dealers. Early in February 1916 the director revealed his misgivings to the new health commissioner, Dr. Haven Emerson, formerly deputy commissioner, who had assumed the position when Goldwater resigned. Emerson, in turn, spoke to Mayor Mitchel. The mayor ordered the commissioner of accounts, Leonard M. Wallstein, to begin an investigation. On 26 May, as a result of evidence collected by Wallstein, veterinarian inspector Dr. Frederic W. Schoneweg, and special investigator William H. Boyle, Brown dismissed several meat inspectors who had allegedly taken bribes from the operators of slaughterhouses. During the same period the city obtained indictments against twelve dealers on the charge of bribery, four of whom were convicted, and it revoked permits for the operation of the businesses in question.[16]

Unorthodox dealers had developed a sophisticated strategy over the years. Lookouts signaled the approach of honest inspectors. Employees then lowered undesirable meat into compartments covered by trap doors. Corrupt officers presented no problems. Therefore, when they appeared, dealers reversed the process: Good meat disappeared and foul meat came out of hiding. For twenty years or more, authorities believed, the practice of bribing inspectors to pass "sleepers"—unfit carcasses—had been a common practice. The money ranged from $50 to $75 a week per man, depending on services rendered. Graft amounted to between $35,000 and $40,000 annually. Schoneweg, posing as a new inspector, gleaned much of this information. When he took up his duties, one of the meat dealers told him: "You ought to get wise." When he inquired further, the man informed him that it was possible "to make a little on the side." Pressing for even more information, he was told: "Don't be foolish; you know what I meant; everybody is getting it."[17]

It was not surprising that inspectors succumbed to temptation, for their annual salaries amounted to only $1,200 to $1,400. Many of them had wives, children, and dependent relatives to support, and they were hard put financially to keep up their responsibilities. The low pay, coupled with the desire of some dealers to palm off inferior goods in return for excess profits, created a natural breeding ground for corruption. Then, too, the chances of being caught seemed slim because the field inspectors were isolated from the central administration.[18]

Along with a reliable staff, Brown needed a receptive public. In Tennessee, Brown single-handedly had launched a program of public health education; in New York, the Bureau of Public Health Education covered this work. The director of that bureau issued publications, planned exhibits and lectures, showed moving pictures, and maintained the departmental library. Nonetheless, other bureau chiefs cooperated closely with him. In July 1915, Brown hastily put together information on food and drug control for release to the press. Some articles dealing with the fish business soon appeared. Alfred W. McCann of the *Globe* took an avid interest in the new bureau director and predicted that he would save the citizens a great deal of money "if the city fathers will give him the men necessary to keep up the pace." The *Herald* gave a similar but less verbose coverage. These beginnings seemed promising to Brown, who remarked: "I think that with proper handling here we can get some interest in the papers, for the people seem to take the same interest in pure food work here as elsewhere, and the publicity bureau of the Department is anxious for all the stuff we can give them."[19]

Brown took advantage of opportunities to inform the public. From 26 December 1915 to 2 January 1916 the Bureau of Food and Drugs and the Bureau of Public Health Education, in conjunction with the Emerson Society of the University Settlement House, sponsored a pure food show. On 27 December the director himself delivered a lecture, "Supervising the Food of Five Million People." In November 1916 the bureau set up an exhibit at the Twenty-second

Regimental Armory as part of a food show sponsored by the New York Retail Grocers' Association. An inspector who was on hand for the occasion explained the methods of inspection, pointed out the waste of food involved in poor handling and shipping, and showed some samples of adulterated food.[20]

Brown thought it only fair that businessmen be provided with information about regulations and that they be given ample time to conform to standards before they were subjected to prosecution. He, therefore, set out to win over legitimate dealers. The Jews, as an ethnic group, presented a challenge, and Brown seemed determined to win their acceptance. "The only way to handle the Jews," he said, "is to get their confidence." He explained that he found this to be imperative:

> As there are 1,250,000 of them in our total population of 5,500,000, they must be handled. So I have already gone to a meeting with one set of push-cart men and expect to go to others. I have also come into contact with, and apparently have the confidence of, the Jews at the head of their social uplift work here, very bright, smart, straight men—and I have begun a little study of the problem—People to whom I have talked say this is the only way of handling these people —it's the way I have always handled any people.[21]

Brown felt confident by August 1915 that he was gaining the cooperation of his "Yiddish friends."

Other businessmen were not neglected, for efforts to maintain good relations with them as well as with the general public were constant. In October 1915 the Bureau of Food and Drugs scheduled a meeting of restaurateurs. Discussion followed the lectures of Brown and his staff. Owners showed genuine interest and commended the bureau for its efforts. A few suggested that stricter enforcement and more drastic action might be desirable in some cases. During December, representatives from the bureau conferred with meat and fish dealers. On 14 February 1917, Brown delivered a lecture at a banquet of the New York Wholesale Grocers' Association on "Functions of a State in Food Control." The same day, Assistant Director Ole Salthe met with the Confectioners and Ice Cream

Manufacturers of New York State and spoke on "The Relation of the Department of Health to Confectioners and Ice Cream Manufacturers." On 14 April, at the Department of Health, the assistant director and staff members presented a program for eighty students from Cornell University on food conditions in general and on poultry and eggs in particular.[22]

Educational activities attracted interest and publicity, but the bureau gained the most attention when it cast a searchlight on wrongdoers and brought them to justice. Enforcement, after all, was the major function of this branch of the Health Department. Under Brown's direction, it did not shirk its responsibilities. Investigators kept up a steady program of inspection, but this aspect of the work went virtually unnoticed except in annual reports which the experts wrote for each other. The public was titillated more by sensationalism than by monotonous routine. Brown took his old campaign technique, which had been perfected in his native state, out of mothballs, breathed new life into it, and stirred the imaginations of cosmopolitan New Yorkers.

With slight alteration, the campaign, as a weapon against illegal practices, functioned well in New York City. In Tennessee, Brown generally waged campaigns during the summer within a limited period of time in a given city or town. In this gigantic port city a campaign was almost constantly under way against some group of food dealers. Frequently the bureau put several in motion at the same time. The overwhelming number of violations by food handlers— whether wholesalers, retailers, restaurateurs, or pushcart vendors— kept the inspection staff overworked. The campaign technique itself retained its former characteristics—sensationalism, careful scrutiny by a number of health officials, and well-publicized arrests and prosecutions.

The complexity of problems presented by the nefarious dealers in New York led Brown to take up "the raid" as a part of his grand strategy. The principal difference in "the raid" and "the campaign" centered on the objectives. The campaign, announced in advance, allowed those who were subjected to it a chance to alter any practices that were in violation of the law or the Sanitary Code before inspectors appeared. The raid, on the other hand, required great secrecy and careful planning after the bureau had learned of violators who wantonly endangered public health. According to Brown, it was "often necessary to make regular raids on certain industries." In such a raid during October 1915, "fifty-six men were detailed to cover food-handling establishments, especially with reference to the use of rotten eggs." As a result the inspectors uncovered fifty violations of the Sanitary Code and condemned about eleven hundred pounds of unfit food that they found in bakeries.[23]

As a novice, Brown gingerly tested public opinion. In July 1915 he began a minor campaign to protect "Summer widowers," being one himself, who were compelled to eat in restaurants because their families were out of the city on vacation. He ordered inspectors to concentrate their work on restaurants in residential districts, checking to see that food was properly handled and prepared.[24] After two months on the job, Brown announced that he had familiarized himself with local conditions and was prepared to direct a vigorous campaign to improve the food supply. He indicated, however, that special consideration would be given to small businessmen:

> Inasmuch as some of the regulations are highly scientific and technical, first offenders, particularly smaller dealers, will be handled with some measure of leniency. After a first warning, however, the bureau will proceed relentlessly against keepers of unclean stores, sellers of unfit foods and other violators of regulations. The bureau will be much more severe in its handling of the larger dealers, who are in a better position to familiarize themselves with the law.[25]

The fish business came under close scrutiny within a month of the warning, and the legendary Fulton Market, through which 90 percent of the supply of the city passed, was not overlooked. Prior to Brown's appointment, "the ordinary fish shipping box was used for the display of fish, foul river water was used for washing purposes, and floors were filthy, and conditions in general bad." During 1915 the situation improved. The director reported that "hearty co-operation was received from the fish dealers themselves." "Old employees," he said, stated that the market was in "better condition than for forty years."[26]

Fish dealers as a group were not lacking in imagination. Health

Department inspectors discovered plain codfish that had been dyed to resemble Alaskan salmon. A New York newspaper gave the following account:

> The codfish were acquiring the glow of sunset in boxes down in cold storage under the Manhattan arches of the Brooklyn Bridge when an inspector of the Health Department routed them out and looked them over with care. On the boxes was the label, "Alaskan Salmon," but inside there were denizens of the Cape Cod neighborhood in various shades of reds and pinks. The top layers of fish were red through and through, then there were layers of a feeble solferino, and last of all layers as white as the flesh of any cod that ever dozed along the coast.[27]

The process involved soaking the fish in pyroligneous acid and then sousing them in Zanzibar red. Plied by energetic hucksters as salmon, the incarnadined cod sold at forty cents a pound instead of ten cents, the going rate for the plain variety.

Raids and campaigns remained common throughout Brown's years in New York, persistently attracting attention to the bureau. A new grading program gained a great deal of publicity during 1916. At the end of May the director announced that he was ordering inspectors, beginning in June, to investigate the conditions in every hotel and restaurant in the city. The survey included not only the premises where food was stored, prepared, and served but also the personal cleanliness of cooks, waiters, and kitchen assistants. As soon as the routine had been completed, owners received a card that showed a rating of good, fair, or bad. In order to obtain the highest grade, a facility had to comply with a list of fifty conditions, twenty-six of which were compulsory. If any one of the twenty-six requirements was not met, the business received a grade of fair or bad.[28]

Although grading was an innovation in New York City, the practice had been established by Brown in Tennessee during 1911. In the big city it stimulated a flurry of excitement. Brown did not require proprietors to display grading cards, but he encouraged patrons to ask to see them and then to eat with assurance or go elsewhere in pursuit of sanitary food. The Times commented that such a policy seemed rather absurd at first thought: "Telling just when the inspectors are coming, and what merits they will reward and what faults they will penalize, is, of course, no way to bring sinners to punishment or to drag exciting scandals into the sight of a shocked and interested public. Having been duly warned, the proprietors of these places will take good care to have everything all right betimes, and if anything hasn't been all right in the past, proof of that fact will be difficult or impossible." The editor praised the wisdom of the health officials and noted, "They are quite justified in thinking that it is not the previous condition of these kitchens that really counts, but their present and future condition. To accomplish that better end the board is using an excellent method."[29]

Initial inspections revealed the need for "a pure food revival," but the restaurant keepers responded well to criticism of their methods. Interestingly enough, a Bowery saloon that served free lunches was the first of its type to receive a "good" rating. "Why do you give away large quantities of bread to these poor men?" one of the inspectors asked the Irish proprietor. "My mother died not long ago," was the noble answer, "and in her will she begged me to give soup, meat, and bread to any man who came in my place of business, provided, of course, that he felt hungry. My back room is a club dining room. Come, look!"[30] Odds were that the owner of the saloon marshaled the homeless men whom he allowed to sleep in the place into a troop of voters for Tammany politicians or one of the ward bosses. Another inspection on a morning following a cold winter night might have revealed surroundings that were not quite so sanitary.

Inspectors graded between four and five hundred restaurants by the end of July. Brown reported that this work had been severely curtailed because his staff had been assisting in efforts to check the poliomyelitis epidemic. These initial inspections showed, however, that restaurants in the city were not measuring up well to requirements. The public seemed ready to panic, and Dr. Bolduan soon issued statements designed to allay fears.[31]

The grading experiment during the summer of 1916 raised the possibility of placing food-handling establishments under a permit plan. The final decision rested with Mayor Mitchel and Commissioner Wallstein. On 30 January 1917 the Board of Health, with the mayor's consent, amended the Sanitary Code, thereby requiring every eating place in New York City to obtain permission from the commissioner of health to stay in business. The provision took effect immediately. By the end of March nearly fifteen thousand proprietors had made application.[32]

Alerting the public to hidden dangers in food remained an objective of the Department of Health. Experts there realized that economic considerations tended to receive highest priority from businessmen. If customers understood the risks involved, dealers might be forced to conform to standards or lose trade. The director of the bureau had this in mind when he began a campaign against exposed food. Each year this unsanitary practice resulted in the condemnation of thousands of pounds of edibles that had been contaminated by flies, dust, and dirt. Dealers at city markets, the pushcart vendors, and the operators of sidewalk stands shared responsibility for this problem.[33]

Brown had a penchant for waging war on flies. With a little imagination it was possible to conjure up horrible visions by considering conditions to be found in most large cities. Lawrence Veiller, a leading authority on housing in New York, had once made the following observation on an alley located in the tenement districts: "Piles of manure, those pest factories which breed uncontrolled the typhoid fly by myriads, frequently overflow into it. Uncollected garbage, in the hot summer months, lies there in decaying heaps. Surface water, slops, wash-tub emptyings, leakage from privies and from stables cover the surface with slime. Old paper, tin cans, rubbish and refuse of every kind are everywhere; huge rats, living and dead, add to the general horror."[34] Only a short flight separated the flies in the alley from the pushcarts, which operated almost exclusively in the tenement districts. Such organizations as the New York Association for Improving Conditions of the Poor had tried to educate the vendors. The average operator, however, made no move to adopt procedures recommended by reformers, which included the expense of covering the carts with glass. Generally scorned, the itinerant peddlers, numbering at least ten thousand, sold food one day and might well be pushing "shoe strings or underwear" the next. On the East Side alone, according to Brown, twenty-seven streets were devoted to pushcart markets. These little conveyances caused a never-ending headache for inspectors who repeatedly examined them, issued warnings, and sometimes prosecuted the operators.[35]

Exposure of food to filth at the city markets also presented problems. In 1877, William H. Rideing, a journalist, had noted that there were ten public markets in New York, not one of them worthy of the amount of business it received. While conditions at the markets had been bad, the approaches to them had been worse. On wet days, so he had written, streets were "sloughs of despair," "ankle-deep in mud." Old vegetable scroungers made frequent rounds, foraging in garbage. The very poor could be seen "poring over a festering heap of decayed stalks and leaves, and raking over each morsel with fixed hungry care."[36] By 1915, changes had been implemented in some of the markets, but they still were far from being free of problems. Washington Market, which had been reconstructed by the city, had become a model of its kind. West Washington Market likewise had undergone pronounced alterations. Brown discovered that the "careless method of covering meat in transit with unclean horse blankets" had been discontinued entirely, refrigerators had been cleaned, and vehicles carrying meat had been rigidly inspected.[37]

In spite of general improvements of city markets over the years, they remained habitats for hoards of flies. This problem at Washington Market received the attention of a special conference of city officials on 24 July 1916. Brown and others thought that screening offered no solution because of the large area of floor space and the volume of business conducted. They decided, as an alternative, to install fans and to keep food on the counters to a minimum. Mrs. F. C. Hogdon, chairman of the Jefferson Market Committee, fired off a letter to the editor of the *Times*. She pointed out that during the previous summer her committee had installed fly traps at the Jefferson Market which were catching flies in "quantities." She suggested that if the doors and windows were screened, the market would be virtually free of the pesky insects. Whatever the advantages of screening, the issue was laid to rest, at least for the time being.[38]

The campaigns and raids that were conducted during 1915 and 1916 involved rather staggering numbers of inspections as well as the destruction of millions of pounds of unwholesome products. The

total of inspections for 1915 was 730,149; figures are not available for
1916. During 1915 the bureau condemned 18,479,275 pounds of food;
in 1916, 12,074,081. Prosecutions were also forthcoming as indicated
in the accompanying table. Figures for 1916 showed an increase in new

Prosecutions	1915	1916
New arrests	4,381	6,223
Number fined	3,133	4,792
Sentences suspended	1,402	1,158
Amount of fines	$33,221	$44,402
Prison sentences	14	15

arrests, fines, and amount of fines collected. Perhaps this indicated
more diligence on the part of inspectors as the result of a tougher
policy toward violators. On the other hand, the figures also revealed
that lawbreakers found security in the immense area of Greater New
York that inspectors had to cover and they risked fines or jail sentences
in spite of the stricter attitudes of the Bureau of Food and Drugs.[39]

The bureau had responsibility for the control of drugs as well
as food. From 1915 to 1917, however, the latter took priority over
the former in spite of the director's personal interest in drug-related
problems. This might be attributed to the size of the drug division,
which included a field force of three inspectors in 1917. The responsibility for drug control in the whole city rested with this limited staff;
nonetheless, a few convictions had been forthcoming. Efforts of this
division to force patent-medicine manufacturers to register with the
Department of Health, however, did not go well. The dealers took
a test case before the courts to determine the constitutionality of
this section of the Sanitary Code. In the appellate division of the
state supreme court, the justices ruled unanimously that "since the
ordinance had not been ratified by the state legislature it was open
to attack on the ground of unreasonableness." The Department of
Health carried the case to the court of appeals, but it remained
unsettled as late as August 1918.[40]

With the entry of the United States into World War I, food
control itself took a back seat to food conservation. Supplying allied
armies and civilian populations helped to drain American stockpiles.

Food conservation was the phrase of the day—not food control. Patriotic Americans felt called upon to do their bit as the activities of Herbert Hoover's federal food administration picked up momentum. New Yorkers considered causes of food waste, and they formed committees; suburbanites grew backyard gardens; ministers preached the gospel of conservation to their congregations; and Camp Fire Girls distributed "household tags" to housewives who pledged themselves to saving food. Meanwhile, Director Brown commented testily that it would be better to stop wasting food than to grow victory gardens. "There is 10 per cent less garbage than New Yorkers threw out two years ago, but," Brown added, "an appalling amount is wasted even now, particularly by more prosperous families."[41]

Mayor Mitchel, a zealous supporter of the war effort, announced the formation of the New York City Food Aid Committee for the purpose of ascertaining the difficulties and needs of citizens there. Perhaps more of a patriotic trapping than a functional organization, the executive committee included George W. Perkins, chairman of the Mayor's Food Committee; Miss Mabel Kittredge, chairman of the Women's Food Committee of the Mayor's Defense Committee; William G. Willcox, one of Brown's neighbors on Staten Island, who was president of the Board of Education; and Brown. The mayor also selected forty-six women to serve as district organizers.[42]

In addition to serving on the New York City Food Aid Committee, Brown geared the work of his inspectors to conservation. During 1917 they made a conscious effort to salvage partially spoiled food shipments. In suitable instances these goods were turned over to charitable organizations for canning. Brown himself published several articles related to conservation, most of which were printed in professional journals, and he delivered papers and lectures on the subject to diverse audiences. He constantly urged shippers to be careful in packing fragile items, and he asked consumers to avoid waste.[43]

Along with the routine responsibilities and patriotic obligations, Brown maintained his contacts with professional organizations and produced a steady stream of scientific publications. Already recognized as one of the country's leading experts on food sanitation as well as public health and agricultural chemistry, he was well established professionally. He regularly attended annual meetings of the American Public Health Association. When in September 1915 the association held its convention at Rochester, New York, the director presented two papers before the general session, one on the grading of milk and the other on the narcotics problem. He also established contacts with other health authorities in New York State. The next year, Brown followed the association to Cincinnati. In 1917 he served as chairman of the food and drug section when the group met in Washington, D.C. Food organizations that were more singular in purpose than the American Public Health Association had the active support of the director. During 1916 he attended a meeting in Philadelphia of health officials from surrounding cities and states. Out of this conclave, with the cooperation of federal officials, the Central Atlantic Food Officials' Association was born. While assisting in the creation of this new society, Brown occasionally appeared at the meetings of the Association of American Dairy, Food and Drug Officials.[44]

Brown continued to think of himself as a professional chemist as well as an expert on food and drug control. In November 1915 he joined his peers in Washington, D.C., for a meeting of the Association of Official Agricultural Chemists. When the American Chemical Society held its second annual exposition at Grand Central Palace in September 1916, he delivered a paper on the chemistry of milk before the food section of the organization. He and another chemist, Clarence V. Ekroth of the Department of Health, also collaborated during 1917 on two articles dealing with the inspection of milk in New York City which appeared in the *Journal of Industrial and Engineering Chemistry*.[45]

From 1915 to 1917 the transplanted Tennessean adjusted well to the metropolis. Once Brown had accustomed himself to his new environment and had gained a reasonably firm control over his employees, he turned to a propaganda program that was designed to win the support of businessmen and ordinary citizens for his work. There were many unorthodox dealers, aided to some degree by unscrupulous inspectors, who remained beyond the pale of his admirers. Against these, Brown used the old campaign technique that he had carried north from Tennessee. When the situation warranted, he and his inspectors raided establishments that were willfully endangering public health. Grading, too, had been one of his innovations in the South. His adoption of this course of action in New York City paved the way for a restaurant permit plan. By 1917, food conservation superseded food control and occupied a considerable amount of his time.

The director did not enjoy the same degree of flexibility in New York as in Tennessee. In the South he had created and enlarged his department and had determined policy; in the North the hierarchy was fixed. He could not enlarge his staff significantly, and standards were outlined in the Sanitary Code. To a limited extent, he determined policy, but all of his work came under the review of the commissioner of health. Brown was above all else a professional. He reveled in the company of the other experts, most of whom, like himself, occupied their positions because of their scores on competitive civil-service examinations. The Department of Health represented a utopia for these scientists, a haven from political trials and tribulations. The term of reform Mayor John P. Mitchel came to an end early in 1918, and the idealistic world of these health experts was shattered. According to the dicta of Tammany Hall, government was the business of politicians. A new mayor, in 1918, set out to rid the city of this strange breed of scientific experts who had invaded the sphere of professional politicians.

7—The Scientist
and Urban Politics, 1918:
Tammany Hall versus the Experts

When 1918 opened in New York City, a battle shaped up between two distinct, sophisticated groups of professionals—the health experts and the politicians. Since the creation of Greater New York City, reformers had fought the Democratic organization for municipal offices because they believed that their own political control of the city was indispensable to the realization of genuinely constructive changes. Both Tammany Hall and the good-government forces courted the naturalized immigrants and second-generation voters. Neither power bloc was able to maintain control of city politics. Weakened by reform campaigns, the machine leaders had become increasingly suspicious of the appearance of any power conglomerates in the city. Therefore, the professional politicians viewed the health-department experts as a threat. By May 1918 the jobs of many scientists were in jeopardy, but Lucius Polk Brown became the special target of the forces led by Mayor John F. Hylan. Before Brown was put to the personal test, however, a major power struggle developed between Tammany politicians and health experts.

After 1898 the Department of Health had become increasingly powerful. The board's authority to draft sanitary regulations having the force of law, the creation of the bureau plan of administration, and the adherence of the health establishment to civil-service regulations infringed on Tammany's domain; practical Democratic politicians regarded government as their personal sphere. During the four years that reformer John P. Mitchel had occupied the mayor's chair, scientific bureaucrats at the Department of Health had entrenched themselves. Therefore, when John Hylan, the Tammany-backed candidate, won the mayoral election of 1917, he launched an attack against the experts that did not end until he had undermined the bureau plan and had obtained the resignation of a number of the administrators, replacing them with his own men. Tammany, however, had not reckoned with the possibility that the experts were capable of launching a strong counteroffensive. The politicians probably expected the scientists to wilt at the first sign of opposition. If this were, indeed, the case, they were sadly mistaken.

The future of both sets of professionals for the next four years hinged on the outcome of the mayoral election of 1917. Ironically, the nonpartisan aspects of the Mitchel administration, which had freed the experts from political tribulations, were the very weaknesses that led to Mitchel's defeat. John Purroy Mitchel had provided reform elements in New York City with a rare interlude for their social experiments. From 1914 to 1918, individuals of diverse socioeconomic classes, ethnic backgrounds, and religions, united by patriotism and nationalism, had crusaded for civic improvement. The reform coalition, therefore, attracted newly arrived immigrants, who were anxious for American acceptance, as well as native-born patricians.[1]

The cement that bound immigrants and patricians was not durable enough, however, to withstand a strong party fight. During his years in office, Mayor Mitchel created a nonpartisan administration that was conducive to Progressive experiments. The *Boston Transcript*, hailing him as "A Courageous American Mayor," noted that he had put into office, or had accompanied into office, a number of "practical idealists."[2] This paradoxical description of Progressive reformers applied especially to those who were ensconced in the Department of Health. Idealistic in their visions for a better world, they were amazingly practical in many of the strategies that they used to obtain results. While enjoying the security afforded them as scientists by the Mitchel administration, some of them nonetheless realized that a defeat for Mitchel in 1917 could eliminate their positions and undermine the bureaucratic structure that they had fashioned for themselves.

Looking for a way to perpetuate this scientific elitism, Deputy Commissioner Haven Emerson urged in 1915 that the "cherished privilege" of New York City mayors to appoint the commissioner of health be discontinued. He insisted on an alteration of policy and law that would make the position permanent. Speaking before the Sixth New York City Conference of Charities and Corrections, he praised the Mitchel administration for its support of public health work: "Thanks to the blessing of non-partisan city administration we can be assured of freedom from political interference with official health work at present. This is not, however, a sufficient safeguard, for nothing less than a Commissioner of Health, assured of suitable compensation and permanent employment, freed from the risk or certainty of replacement with each change of city administration, will permit of that confidence."[3] S. S. Goldwater, who served for a time as commissioner of health under Mitchel, concurred with Emerson's opinion that the department had remained free of political interference.[4]

Even though politics had remained a secondary element, the health commissioners gave Mitchel their support. Emerson, on one occasion, forwarded Mitchel a copy of a speech that he was planning to deliver at Carnegie Hall. He suggested to the mayor that if he wished for him "to take another angle," he should inform him no later than the morning of the day on which the speech was to be given.[5] Unfortunately, the experts at the Department of Health had no guarantee that this type of political-bureaucratic relationship could be sustained. Emerson's suggestion that the position of the commissioner be made permanent had gained no legal ground. Therefore, the health bureaucrats found themselves in a precarious position; they could take solace only in the faint hope that Mitchel would be reelected.

In scientific terms, for every action there is always an equal and opposite reaction. The implications of Newton's Third Law could well be applied to Mitchel's career. His meteoric rise to political stardom was followed by an equally meteoric plummet to earth, figuratively and literally. The ascent began when Mitchel agreed, during George McClellan's tenure as mayor, to serve as an aid to the corporation counsel who was then investigating the municipal corruption that involved borough president John F. Ahearn of Manhattan. Making use of the experience and acquaintances from this position and of that which came with his service as commissioner of accounts, Mitchel, who was then about thirty, became a candidate for president of the Board of Aldermen in 1909. Backed by a combination of Republicans, the Citizens Union, and the Committee of One Hundred, he placed himself above his inherited ties to the Democratic party. When Mayor William J. Gaynor was attacked by a would-be assassin in 1910, Mitchel, as president of the Board of Aldermen, became acting mayor for a time. In 1913 he accepted a federal appointment to be Collector of the Port of New York. This did not last long, however, for in the same year, after much difficulty, he became the compromise candidate of the Fusionists, supplanting George McAneny and Charles S. Whitman. He eventually received the endorsement of the Independents, the Republicans, and political gadfly William Randolph Hearst.[6]

On election day 1913, Mitchel defeated the Tammany candidate, Edward E. McCally, by 121,000, piling up the largest number of votes since the creation of Greater New York. This freakish victory was brought on by a number of factors. Mayor Gaynor had died, depriving Tammany of a candidate who had some support from reformers; their candidate was virtually unknown; and the governor, Tammany-backed William Sulzer, had been impeached, further tarnishing the image of the city's political machine. This election marked the high point of Mitchel's career.[7]

Having ridden to victory without benefit of a party organization, the new mayor had little appreciation for political niceties. Indeed, so scornful was he of the usual vote-getting tactics that he soon alienated many old supporters. He made the following unwise remark when asked by a friendly reporter to comment on a charge made by his opponents that he had socially prominent friends: "Is that an issue? Most of my friends are not in that group. Some are. As to them, I hardly know how to answer, unless—unless I tell them if they don't like my friends they can go to hell."[8] Such comments clearly demonstrated the arrogance that typified his public image.

Not only did the Mitchel administration lack a charismatic politician, but also its record failed to show any dynamic improvement over those of its predecessors. Edwin R. Lewinson, one of Mitchel's biographers, delivered the following verdict: "The Mitchel Administration was beset by many of the pitfalls which hampered other reform administrations of the period. It was honest and well-meaning, but it accomplished little and it failed to win popular support." Gustavus Myers had taken a different tack in campaign propaganda published during the election year. He called the Mitchel administration "one of wholesome tendencies and accomplishments." He added: "It is not contended that evils have entirely disappeared, but at any rate the base, ignoble practices and the repellant incompetence of past 'boss' rule have been much supplanted by improved methods, expert judgment, technical experience, a higher tone, and good spirit."[9]

Americans have never been particularly impressed by expertise and high-toned politics. New Yorkers were no exception. By 1917 the citizens of Gotham wanted a change. A mayor without oratorical skills and machine-making abilities could not play on the heartstrings of a fickle people. William L. Chenery, in an article for the *Atlantic Monthly* in 1924, made the following assessment: "The people of New York do not expect too much of politics. Time and again, they have revolted against Tammany's wickedness only to find that a Whig, a Reformer, a Republican, or a Coalitionist was not more to their taste." While Mitchel refused to provide showmanship for the New Yorkers, Tammany did not. According to Chenery,

> Tammany Hall has never been radical, but espouses popular causes. Moreover, since the early decades of the nineteenth century it has been the professed friend of aliens in a city constantly being resettled by immigrants. It has had singularly attractive social and charitable features and its leaders, from one generation to another, have understood the average man. The "human equation" has had few mysteries for them. Most important of all, Tammany has made a business of politics.[10]

The brains of Tammany, Grand Sachem Charles Francis Murphy, set out to find a satisfactory party solution to the "human equation" in 1917. Murphy, without a doubt, was one of the unique bosses in

American history—the politician's politician, but also open-minded to reform. As boss, he was, according to some observers, "a sort of king or thane," "the embodiment of the tribe." During his rule, city government improved, and Tammany became less disreputable. One journalist explained the change this way: "This is largely because Murphy's conception of the tribe grew with the years—it had come to include Jews and even Protestants. It had expanded to include the State." Described by contemporaries as "a relaying point between the people and officialdom," he kept his ear attuned to the tempos of the times. Because reform occupied several beats, he paid it some attention.[11]

When Murphy searched for a candidate in 1917, he took several factors into account. First, William Randolph Hearst had parted company with Mitchel, apparently over appointments. His presses could be put to good use for Tammany. Second, the politics of the moment seemed to demand a Brooklyn man for the candidacy. Since the creation of Greater New York, Tammany had sought to cross the bridge and take over the Brooklyn Democratic organization. Until 1909, Boss Patrick McCarren had prevented the absorption of his machine by Tammany. He died that year, however, and John Henry McCooey was elected chairman of the Kings County Democratic Executive Committee. A Brooklyn man as candidate for mayor would appease both McCooey and Hearst and would tie the Brooklyn machine more firmly to Tammany. Third, a man who was free from the direct taint of Tammany Hall and bossism would possess considerable advantage over one who was identified exclusively with the Manhattan machine.[12]

A compromise candidate finally emerged to satisfy all the political demands of the moment. Alfred E. Smith apparently wanted the nomination, but Murphy persuaded him to await the gubernatorial year of 1918. Smith accepted this argument but refused to acquiesce in a Hearst candidacy. Therefore, Murphy, Smith, Big Tom Foley—as a Smith supporter and leader of the Lower East Side district—and Hearst decided that John F. Hylan would be a desirable candidate. He was not associated with Murphy; they had not met prior to his selection. As a Brooklynite and a friend of Hearst's, he pleased Boss McCooey. Before Hylan received the nomination, Murphy talked the

the choice over with his Brooklyn counterpart. According to one account, the following exchange took place:

> Murphy reportedly met with "Uncle John" McCooey, the pudgy little boss of Brooklyn, and asked him: "Is Hylan a man we can trust and do business with?"
>
> "He certainly is," Uncle John replied. "Do you want to meet him?"
>
> "No," said Murphy, "I want you to ram him down my throat."[13]

"Red Mike" Hylan, an agreeable six-foot red-head, could have been the principal character in a Horatio Alger story. Portrayed as the barefoot boy from the Catskills, he had the makings of an American folk hero. At the tender age of nineteen, he had left the mountain farm, gone to New York City, and landed a job on the Brooklyn Elevated Railroad. Working on the elevated by day and studying law at night, he eventually passed the bar examinations. Dabbling in local Democratic politics led to his candidacy for a judgeship in the municipal court during 1905. He lost the election, but Mayor McClellan made him a magistrate. By 1914 he had become a county judge through appointment. His subsequent election to that post in 1915 by a large majority brought him to the attention of Murphy and McCooey. When a reporter asked how he had gotten into politics, Hylan answered promptly: "I walked in." He possessed only average intelligence, but the Democratic machine did not need a genius. His complacency and subservience suited Tammany.[14]

Meanwhile, after much soul-searching, Mitchel decided that he would seek reelection. Ironically, he became a victim of one of the good-government reforms—the direct primary. With no hope of any support from the Democratic party, he decided to enter the Republican primary. In a close election that involved irregularities and a recount, he lost to William M. Bennett. By this time, Mitchel had not even the shreds of a connection with any party organization, but he entered the election as an Independent, supported by reform elements. With three candidates already in the field—Hylan, Bennett, and Mitchel—the Socialists nominated one of their outstanding

leaders, Morris Hillquit, who hoped to capitalize on antiwar sentiment.[15]

Prospects for Mitchel were not good; no better were the chances
that the reformers he had placed in the municipal establishment
would survive his defeat. As a mouthpiece of Tammany, Hylan made
clear to the experts what they could expect if the Democrats triumphed
in the November election. As early as September he spoke out against
charitable foundations, which he labeled a menace to the city, to
schools, and to health. Attacking the "aristocracy of experts," he
associated them with the Nietzschean "Superman" concept. Health
Commissioner Haven Emerson received particular attention as a
pawn of the foundations. Hylan singled out for criticism Emerson's
advice during the poliomyelitis epidemic of 1916. The health
commissioner had urged people to get their children out of town.
Quite correctly, Hylan pointed out that tenement dwellers were in
no position to act on such advice.[16] If the health experts realized
their vulnerability, they had no choice except to support Mitchel;
Tammany Hall certainly offered them no recourse. Instead of a retreat
for scientists, the Department of Health was viewed by Tammany
as a reservoir of jobs for loyal party workers.

Election day 1917 proved to be a dreary one for reformers.
Mitchel, who had been swept into office by the largest majority since
1897, went out under a Hylan avalanche which exceeded his vote of
four years earlier. W. M. Houghton of the *Tribune* rendered a
fitting analysis of the Mitchel disaster. He said that the mayor was
defeated "because the good citizens of this town swallowed what
Hearst said about him, that he was a frivolous tango-dancer, that he
was a social climber and snob, that he was a friend of the 'plunder-
bund,' a little brother of the rich, an arrogant ally of Rockefeller."[17]
Smarting from this humiliating defeat, Mitchel, always a strong
supporter of the war effort, enlisted in the Air Corps. Already dead
politically, he completed his demise when he fell out of an airborne
single-seater training plane.

The New York City press had generally favored Mitchel's
candidacy. When it became apparent that Tammany had returned
to power, the newspapers were not enthusiastic about the prospects
for an administration headed by Hylan. An editorial in the *World*

lamented: "Tammany has come back to power. By the irony of fate it has come back to power under the most unfit, incompetent candidate for Mayor that it has nominated since consolidation." The *Globe* took comfort in the fact that Hearst would gain little, adding, "Tammany hasn't often done all the fighting when it has won, but it has always got all the booty." The *Post* editorial grieved: "What cuts deepest is the thought that all the fine work done under the Mitchel administration during the four years past seems to have been trampled upon by the city." Hearst's *American* chided the other newspapers for changing their attitude toward Hylan after the election, although it hardly seemed that they had done so, and promised that Hylan would justify his wife's faith—that the city would be proud of him.[18]

As soon as the fog that accompanied the election returns lifted from the heads of reformers, they began to wonder what action Hylan would take. When the mayor-elect hinted that the victory he had won might have been a mandate to cut city expenditures, the *Times* pragmatically suggested that the civil service might keep some jobs out of Tammany's clutches. Hylan soon attacked the Bureau of Municipal Research, charging that it was practically maintained by the Rockefellers and those who were in sympathy with them. His initiative apparently startled Tammany Hall. Charles Francis Murphy returned from a vacation to talk with Hylan.[19]

Stark realities of the November election soon settled down on reformers in New York. Professor Charles-Edward A. Winslow of Yale University, an ardent advocate of public health reform, challenged the New York Women's City Club to protect the Department of Health: "We have the best municipal Health Department in the world, and what has the Women's City Club done to see that it will be continued? We have a new Mayor—have you been to ask him if he is going to put as good a man in the Health Board as Haven Emerson? If you have not, as a City Club you should have done so. You may be sure that there have already been many people to ask about getting the position."[20] The warning came none too soon. The new administration had already taken steps to oppose the selection of thirty district health officers whose salaries had not been included in the city budget of 1918. Charles I. Stengel, who managed

Hylan's campaign in Brooklyn, appeared before the Civil Service Commission and protested their drawing up a list of eligible candidates.[21]

The choice of a commissioner of health began to rest heavily on the minds of reform-oriented New Yorkers. In an editorial, the *Times* reminded Hylan that his appointment should be above all the considerations of party politics and still farther above the thought of "patronage" or "the organization." Whatever conspiracy might be afoot, the Citizens Union, led by William Jay Schieffelin, trained a suspicious eye on the Hylan administration and waited to see whether to support it or to fight it.[22]

Hylan announced the name of his new commissioner of health on 15 January. Dr. J. Lewis Amster—who was president of the Bronx County Medical Society, a loyal worker for the Democrats, and one of Murphy's cronies—received the appointment. No immediate repercussions followed. In early April, however, Hylan launched the first phase of his assault on the Department of Health. He sent Amster a letter telling him to remove seven of the bureau directors. Apparently the mayor chose to recognize the legitimacy of only the old Bureau of Sanitary Inspection and the Bureau of Registry and Statistics; both had gone out of existence with the reorganization that had taken place in the Department of Health between 1910 and 1914. An unwilling party, Amster, who was not sure of the desirability of such a move, suggested that Hylan have the Civil Service Commission and the commissioner of accounts, David Hirschfield, investigate the legality of the creation of the new bureaus. Then, he promised, after the findings were submitted to the corporation counsel, to act according to the legal opinion.[23]

This action marked the beginning of a major power struggle between two highly organized groups whose interests conflicted. Public health had become a matter for scientifically trained experts; politics represented the domain of another group of professionals. The New York City Department of Health occupied a branch of municipal government, and from a professional political perspective, the jobs it provided should have been available for patronage. The scientists who had entered municipal government as health reformers, however, believed that their sphere should be protected by civil-service regulations from the recurring political storms of passing administrations. Politicians and scientists, unwilling to compromise without a fight, drew their lines and summoned their warriors. Distinctions between the two groups blurred, however, in the heat of battle. At times it became difficult to separate the professional scientist from the professional politician. Furthermore, fissures developed in what had appeared to be united fronts. Scientists, it seemed, could be aspiring politicians as well, and politicians were not always united in purpose, especially in a metropolis where problems of borough sovereignty beset machine politics.

Under the guise of legality, the probe to eradicate the directorships began on 9 April. James E. MacBride, the Tammany chairman of the Civil Service Commission, made no secret of his opinion that the bureau system was "manifestly improper." He promised to recommend that it be discontinued. Among the first witnesses to be called were Commissioner Amster; Lucius Polk Brown; Dr. Frank Krause, sanitary superintendent; Dr. William F. Guilfoy, registrar of the Bureau of Vital Statistics; and Dr. Louis Harris, director of the Bureau of Preventable Diseases.[24]

For the most part, individuals like Brown, who were recognized as experts in the field of public health, headed these bureaus. They included: Dr. S. Josephine Baker of the Bureau of Child Hygiene; Bolduan, Public Health Education; Harris, Preventable Diseases; Guilfoy, Vital Statistics; Krause, Sanitary Bureau; Dr. William H. Park, Bureau of Laboratories; and Dr. Robert J. Wilson, Bureau of Hospitals. Of this group, Brown was the most recent employee of the Department of Health. The others were veterans of many years, some having been employed in the 1890s. The newest director in the department, recently appointed by Hylan to the Bureau of General Investigation, was Dr. Frank J. Monaghan, the mayor's personal physician.[25]

To attack the legitimacy of the bureaus seemed, on the surface, to be a master stroke by Hylan, for this strategy helped to conceal the more ominous side of the matter. The bureau plan of administration had been debated within the Department of Health itself, but Hylan made it appear that the experts were jeopardizing efficient health administration merely to perpetuate their own establishment. Former

Commissioner Goldwater in 1914 had noted the weaknesses of the bureau plan. To deal with major difficulties, he established Health District Number 1 on an experimental basis and soon reported that it had much to commend itself. Chamberlain Bruère summarized the advantages of the experiment in a report, "New York City's Administrative Progress—1914–1916." This district arrangement apparently made the health administration somewhat more flexible than the bureau plan alone; it also afforded a more personal approach.[26]

Tammany officials, dragged along by the momentum of political bungling, set out to use the Department of Health's own experiment to eliminate the bureau plan. Attempting to cast the experts as impersonal scientists operating in a sterile world aloof from the problems of the masses, they pitted themselves as the champions of the citizens. This strategy, however, failed to hide their sinister objectives. The abolition of the bureau plan would naturally result in the elimination of many civil-service classifications. The need would then arise for new civil-service positions under new classifications. This meant new jobs to be filled by new appointees—Tammany appointees. In an editorial, the *Times* incisively cut through the cloudy morass of explanations: "Back of all this solemn feinting lies, presumably, the immortal Tammany doubt: Is it legal for anybody not a Tammany devotee to hold office under the City Charter?"[27]

The opinion of the *Times* seemed justified, especially in light of the veil of secrecy that had been cast over the proceedings of the Civil Service Commission. When representatives of several civic organizations arrived at the Municipal Building to sit in on the hearings, they were turned away because, according to MacBride, the hearings represented a "private inquiry" and only those who had been "invited" could attend. Invitations went only to witnesses. If reform groups had any illusions about what the Hylan administration was up to, such secrecy alerted them to the political realities. They began mobilizing for the siege. The New York City Woman Suffrage party responded quickly, called on the mayor, and asked him to reconsider any interest that he might have in abolishing the Bureau of Child Hygiene. The Women's Municipal League also condemned the investigation. In a public statement the members pointed out that the city would surely lose the services of trained experts if the citizens did not rise up in indignant protest. They also argued that the bureaus were not "fads and frills" of the Mitchel administration but had originated in the days of Mayors Gaynor and McClellan.[28]

Still attempting to maintain a precarious balance between Hylan and the reformers, Amster persuaded the physicians of the city to await the outcome of the investigation before taking action. Reports had it that if the bureaus were deemed illegal, the mayor would' order them abolished and would divide the work among the assistant sanitary superintendents of the five boroughs. On 13 April, representatives of the medical societies, disregarding Amster's arguments, joined those from labor organizations, social agencies, and the Bar Association to discuss the advisability of instituting a taxpayers' suit to compel the Civil Service Commission to produce all records and papers connected with the hearings. Attending were such prominent citizens as Dr. Lee K. Frankel, chairman of the Committee of Twenty-one; J. H. Larson, secretary of the New York Milk Committee; and Ernest Bohm, secretary of the Central Federated Union. This meeting came on the same day that MacBride added a new dimension to the secret inquiry. What had been an investigation of the legitimacy of the seven bureaus that were not specifically mentioned in the charter suddenly became a search for graft in the Department of Health.[29]

Reformers grew increasingly concerned over the plight of the bureaus. On 15 April the presidents of the New York medical societies joined with Dr. Abraham Jacobi, "the dean of the medical profession," in a public statement to citizens. They pointed out the dangers involved in tampering with the health administration. At the same time, Dr. Lee K. Frankel made repeated and unsuccessful efforts to see the mayor. The suspicious silence emanating from the Hylan camp led the New York State Consumers' League, the Cooper Union Forum, and the New York Child Labor Committee to add their strength to those who opposed Hylan.[30]

As the struggle intensified, outsiders contributed to the general confusion. Representatives of the American Public Health Association and the American Medical Association wrote to Hylan, telling him that it would be a calamity to abolish the Bureau of Public Health Education. Charles V. Chapin, the noted health authority in Providence, Rhode Island, sent the mayor a similar warning. The federal government also took a dim view of Hylan's investigation. As a port of entry, New York was so important that the government officials saw this as a possible threat to national security, particularly during wartime. On 28 April the surgeon general, Rupert Blue, sent Hylan a telegram, urging him not to curtail activities of the Bureau of Public Health Education.[31]

Working conditions at the Department of Health itself became difficult. Dr. William H. Park, director of the Bureau of Laboratories, urged that any reorganization be made speedily because it was hard for employees to function in such an uncertain situation. Meanwhile Commissioner Amster expressed his concern that the efficiency of the department was being impaired. He also announced that none of the bureaus would be "curtailed" while he was in office and that if they were, he planned to resign. Termination of his services was soon forthcoming. On 29 April, Amster submitted his resignation after an unsuccessful interview with Hylan. He had warned the mayor that if the chaos continued, the federal government would surely intervene, and the mayor had replied: "I do not give a darn for these Federal Governmental letters or letters from other people who are interested in public health education. As long as I am Mayor of the City of New York the Health Department will be run as I see fit." The former commissioner reported later that the mayor had demanded that he remove Goldwater and Jacobi from the Medical Advisory Council. Jacobi was the father-in-law of George McAneny of the Times, who had opposed Hylan politically. Goldwater, it seemed, was guilty of being a "highbrow" and a "holdover" from the previous administration. When the letter of resignation reached Hylan, he responded angrily: "I have just received by messenger your resignation as Commissioner of the Department of Health. It gives me great pleasure to accept the same." He also charged Amster with lack of executive ability in allowing graft and special interests to influence his department. The mayor assured Amster that his resignation would not alter policy.[32]

The mayor now had a full-fledged rebellion on his hands. With the resignation of his own appointee, a friend of Murphy's, on his desk, he faced a united group of scientists who were supported by major reform organizations in New York City, to say nothing of interested outsiders, including federal officials. The motley crew of supporters that Hylan mustered had no such claims to prestige. They included political hangers-on and letter writers who, for the most part, chose to remain anonymous. On 19 April the mayor received a communication signed Taxpayer. The unidentified author urged Hylan not to let the socialists, reformers, politicians, and medical profession interfere with his "timely efforts to reorganize the Department of Health." The writer called the department "a nest for breeding socialists, etc., and making Directors, Chiefs of Divisions, Supervisors, etc., and endless red tape." Another anonymous letter to Amster's successor denounced the department's pretensions of saving lives while supporting birth control, an interesting argument in a city overflowing with prolific Catholics and Jews.[33]

Faced with the gauche independence of Hylan, Tammany may have gotten more than it had bargained for in the new mayor. No doubt the tribesmen would enjoy any sweet morsels of patronage that Hylan could throw their way if he were successful in uprooting the experts from the Department of Health. Boss Murphy, however, had a reputation for circumspection. Having once commented that public health was above politics, he certainly had no desire to be connected with well-publicized scandals and intrigues. Nonetheless, when the mayor attacked the Department of Health, Tammany Hall could not escape involvement. The clumsiness with which Hylan and his grasping lieges pawed at the department could only be scorned by such sophisticates as Alfred E. Smith and Boss Murphy.

The outraged demands by the civic, labor, and medical organizations did not go unnoticed by leading Democrats at Tammany Hall. Smith, president of the Board of Aldermen, returned from a vacation during the health crisis. When he was asked by reporters if he would look into the investigation by the mayor, he laughingly replied that all he had time to do was to shake hands. Rumor had it that prominent Democrats were concerned, nonetheless, about the repercussions. On 20 April, Smith visited MacBride, and soon a report was issued that the hearings henceforth would be open to the public. Smith also revealed that the preliminary report recommended the abolition of the Bureau of Public Health Education because it was "useless." Dr.

S. S. Goldwater, who had organized the bureau, immediately offered the opinion that such action would be a mistake.[34]

The grand sachem viewed the situation as serious enough to warrant his return from a vacation. Murphy arrived in New York at the end of April—after spending several weeks at French Lick Springs, Indiana—just in time to learn of Amster's resignation. Murphy told reporters that he was "perfectly satisfied" with the Hylan administration. When asked how he felt about efforts by District Attorney Edward Swann to clean up New York City, however, he snapped: "There is nothing to clean up here. If Mr. Swann thinks the town is not clean he ought to get busy and go out and find the unclean spots."[35]

The resignation of Amster and the return of Murphy marked the end of the first phase of the political war on the health experts. Actually, Hylan, at this point, had not gained much ground. The investigation had brought on reams of undesirable publicity for Tammany; the efficiency of the Department of Health had been impaired; and the Bureau of Child Hygiene had its budget cut by $105,000 after MacBride misrepresented one of Dr. Baker's reports. Dr. Bolduan of Public Health Education, choosing to leave rather than fight, submitted his resignation in early May. Another bureau, Food and Drugs, had been mentioned by MacBride in connection with graft. As the second phase of the attack began, corruption in the bureaus, not their legitimacy, became the main target. Maligned by MacBride, the director of the Bureau of Food and Drugs took up the challenge. A gentleman from the South, Brown considered the accusations to be an attack on his personal honor.[36]

The second phase began with the appointment of a new health commissioner and the exaggerated emphasis on corruption. As soon as Amster resigned, the mayor appointed Royal S. Copeland to the post. The new commissioner, an ophthalmologist, fell into the category of an "expert." Some strange quirk caused his medical mind to bend toward politics. Dr. Frank Crane, writing for a city newspaper, called the mayor's appointment a suspicious one. He added: "Copeland is no politician, understands not the devious art of getting elected, and is just a plain, efficient medical man, with dangerous symptoms of being an expert, even a highbrow." Crane misjudged

Copeland. Outwardly he might have been a physician, but inside him there beat the heart of a politician who had gained previous experience as mayor of Ann Arbor, Michigan, from 1901 to 1903.[37]

When Copeland assumed his new post at the Department of Health, he received several letters from well-wishers. One such individual outlined the reasons that Amster had failed. He mentioned the opposition of the former commissioner to the borough plan of administration and his relationship with the directors. Amster, described as "the spineless man," allegedly met on the day of his appointment with the directors and gave all of them cigars; the writer did not except Dr. Baker. The correspondent did not have a particularly high regard for any of the directors but Park. He called Brown "a fossil" and Bolduan "a joke," and he argued that Harris received too much pay. As for Dr. Baker, she was a friend of Haven Emerson's.[38]

The preliminaries of the second phase of the war on experts soon ended, and the real action began. MacBride wrote to Copeland on 30 April, singling out Lucius Polk Brown for attack. He charged that Brown had shown favoritism toward the Borden Milk Company and William J. Schieffelin & Company, a drug firm with origins in the eighteenth century. He insisted that Leonard M. Wallstein, the paid agent of Schieffelin's Citizens Union, was one of the chief organizers of propaganda to block his investigation. He further alleged that Brown had advocated the passage of a bill by the state legislature that would lower the standard of milk—all this in addition to allowing corruption to flourish in his bureau. MacBride grossly exaggerated the extensiveness of graft. The district attorney managed to obtain indictments against only three employees: Harold J. Keen, T. Spencer Duignan, and Alexander Leibe were charged with bribery and extortion. This, however, certainly did not mean that the director had knowingly allowed corruption to exist.[39]

Brown, Wallstein, and Schieffelin issued denials by the next day. Wallstein, who responded first, expressed the sentiments of them all: "MacBride's vile mouthings do not merit a reply. He apparently fails to recognize the distinction between the tolerance which the public shows to demagogic addresses of this sort, which they expect from people of his kind in the course of a campaign, and what should be the serious utterances of an individual, however unfitted, who holds an important office." Agnes De Lima and Mrs. Edward S. Van Zile, secretary and director, respectively, of the Women's Municipal League, protested the "inaccuracies" of the summary of the testimony given by MacBride. Hylan, meanwhile, urged Copeland to pursue a "fearless" investigation.[40]

On 1 May, just after Copeland took over at the Department of Health, the following demoralizing order from the mayor appeared in the *Staff News*: "All complaints of a criminal nature coming to your department about employees in the City government, signed or unsigned, are to be forwarded to the Police Commissioner at Police Headquarters, so that detectives may be assigned and the violators of the law brought to the bar of justice. All complaints not of a criminal nature, bearing upon the administrative affairs of the department, must be investigated by the respective Department head."[41]

The next day, with the compliance of Hylan, Copeland, who had never met Brown, suspended him. He claimed that if the director had not replied to charges against him, he would not have been punished. The commissioner promised Brown his "day in court," with the opportunity to make explanations. In order that he not be distracted from his duties while preparing for the hearing, Copeland relieved Brown, without pay, until the Board of Health could act on the matter. Meanwhile, former Commissioner Amster revealed that Hylan had insisted earlier that he suspend Brown. The assistant district attorney, however, thought this inadvisable because of the useful information being provided by the director. Several bureau heads came under fire, but no others were suspended. Copeland indicated that he might take over the Public Health Education from Bolduan and possibly even the Division of Industrial Hygiene of the Bureau of Preventable Diseases.[42]

Once Brown had been suspended, he had no doubt that Hylan and Copeland were after his scalp. He promptly hired one of the most prominent lawyers in the city, George Gordon Battle, and began the preparation of a defense. With the reform elements already up in arms because of the attack on the bureau plan, Brown and Battle had little difficulty obtaining the support of the "Mitchelites." To be on the safe side, however, Dr. Carl E. McCombs of the Bureau of Municipal Research, then headed by Charles A. Beard, drafted a form letter to be sent to prominent social and civic leaders. Outlining the accomplishments of the deposed director, he asked for their support.[43]

The preparation of a defense ran into snags. Copeland did not present Brown with a list of specific charges until 28 May. The document received by the director accused him of "neglect of duty, inefficiency, and incompetency." Eleven printed pages in length, it contained only one specification with nine subheads, much of which was repetitive. Essentially Copeland blamed Brown for delegating responsibilities to subordinates; failing to suggest amendments to the Sanitary Code; supporting a bill in the state legislature that would have lowered the quality of milk sold in the city; attending professional conventions, which absented him from New York City; and devoting time to personal activities while on the job. All of this alleged misconduct had occurred prior to the time when Copeland became commissioner.[44]

Faced with these hazy charges, Brown and Battle concentrated on gathering endorsements from acquaintances of the director while drafting a response to each of the complaints. His supporters included not only the Mitchelites but also practically every major health and medical organization in New York and some at the national level, along with food and drug experts throughout the country. An amazingly tight-knit group, these professionals rallied to the aid of their peer. The New York Academy of Sciences and the New York section of the American Chemical Society came out in his defense on 10 May. The AMA *Journal* lashed out at the Hylan administration on 25 May, after having earlier expressed its low opinion of the "private inquiry." Brown himself remained in communication with Dr. Arthur J. Cramp of the Propaganda Department of the AMA. He also kept the American Public Health Association informed of new developments.[45]

Several experts on food and drug control at the state and federal level rose to Brown's defense. Among these were his old friends Harvey W. Wiley and W. D. Bigelow; George H. Adams, chief inspector of the Eastern District for the Department of Agriculture; and Dr. William C. Woodward, district health officer of Washington, D.C. From the states the following added their praise: Charles D. Howard, the state analyst at Concord, New Hampshire; Robert M. Allen, then living in New York City but formerly head of the Food and Drug Division of the Kentucky Agricultural Experiment Station; and William M. Allen, state food and oil chemist of North Carolina.[46]

Friends in Tennessee also expressed support for Brown. H. H. Klein, deputy commissioner of accounts, had drawn the southerners into the turmoil when he wrote to Dr. Perry Bromberg of Nashville on 7 May, asking him to reveal whether it was true that Brown had left the state under a cloud. Bromberg replied that indeed this was not true—that as a matter of record, he had left much to the regret of civic organizations, medical societies, and elected officials. The Nashville physician added that although he did not know what circumstances had prompted the removal of Brown from office in New York, the general feeling in Tennessee was that the director was the victim of political intrigue.[47]

After this incident, Brown asked Tennessee Governor Tom C. Rye for an endorsement, which was immediately forthcoming. Rye noted: "Your unimpeachable record in the office in Tennessee at a time of political distraction is one of the well known facts of recent political history." The secretary of the Tennessee Board of Health, Dr. Olin West, also sent a letter to aid Brown, as did Dr. S. S. Crockett, who had worked to secure the passage of food and drug legislation in the state. The troubled director wrote to his brother Percy at the end of June, asking him to secure the signatures of prominent citizens in Nashville on his behalf. C. R. Frazier, a friend of Brown's at the *Nashville Tennessean and American*, wrote to the director that he could have gotten the names of "practically every man in the city of Nashville if time had permitted." The *Tennessean and American* kept state residents posted on the situation until it was finally resolved.[48]

Moves by the Hylan administration indicated that it was hard put to trump up credible charges against Brown. The letter to Bromberg represented a desperate move. Furthermore, the delay in registering complaints against Brown suggested confusion. When charges were finally released at the end of May, they were not directed toward graft and corruption as initially indicated. The administration also fumbled with the matter of a public hearing. When Copeland released the charges, he informed Brown that he would be granted only a hearing instead of a public trial and that he would not be allowed to call witnesses. The commissioner set the date for 2 June at the exhibition hall of the Department of Health, 139 Centre Street.[49]

The Board of Health consisted of three members, but Copeland was the medium through which the Hylan administration worked. Richard Enright, the police commissioner and a Hylan appointee, remained almost a nonentity on the board. Dr. Leland Cofer, health officer of the Port of New York and the only man on the board who was untainted by Hylanism, took issue with the decision to give Brown only a hearing. He explained: "I believe in a thorough and open investigation and the rendering of a nonpartisan decision. My mind is entirely open on the matter. The question of the kind of trial Dr. Brown was to receive was never brought up at a meeting of the Board of Health where I was present."[50]

Presenting formal charges on 28 May and scheduling the hearing for 2 June gave Brown little time to prepare formal responses. This ploy, however, backfired. The director requested an extension of time, and Copeland, under attack by the press, changed the date to 10 June and promised that the hearing would be open to all interested parties. Legally, Copeland was required to give Brown nothing more than a hearing. The director, however, demanded a public trial and the right to call witnesses. Under municipal guidelines, Copeland could have granted his request. On 10 June, Brown sent a scathing eleven-page typewritten letter to Copeland, questioning his motives. He charged that after his suspension there "ensued a ransacking of department records, and an inquisition of department employees, continuous from that time to this, for the purpose either of supplying a support for Commissioner MacBride's charges, or of furnishing ground for others." Brown added: "This inquisition forced a new abandonment; for Commissioner MacBride's charges were void of proof; they were confuted, rather than supported, by the proof at hand; and I felt secure upon your unqualified promise that public and tested proof alone would be accepted in support of those or any charges which might be produced against me."[51]

The director denounced Copeland for having retracted his promise that witnesses could be called and all charges publicly aired.

"The proof upon which you act is unknown to me," Brown wrote. "I can only surmise it, as it has not been imparted or identified to me. It is not to be tested by me. I may not know whether it is irresponsible back-stairs gossip, or the malice of an unscrupulous enemy, or the self-interest of a prospective successor." Brown argued that strict compliance with provisions of the City Charter afforded him nothing more than "a barren ceremonial." He pointed out to Copeland that the procedure for the hearing was not his exclusive privilege and informed him that he had sent copies of this particular letter to the other two members of the Board of Health. Under fire, the commissioner of health had again rescheduled the hearing, this time to 5 July, whereupon he left town for a vacation.[52]

When the hearing was finally held on 5 July, Dr. Copeland, who was responsible for conducting the session, appeared in his characteristic bright plumage, set off by a vest with white piping. The more somber Brown and his lawyer submitted a comprehensive brief, carefully responding to every known accusation. The director argued that he had carefully supervised his personnel and that the delegation of authority to trusted subordinates was a mark of a good administrator. To the charge that he had failed to suggest revisions for the Sanitary Code, Brown responded that this was "deliberate" because of his personal belief, which was "well known to and not disapproved" by his superiors. He pointed out that it had been the policy of state food administrators to write definitions and standards, using them as a guide, not as hard and fast rules. He added that adoption of standards by small governmental units without federal compliance only complicated trade. Brown admitted that he had supported the Wicks bill, which would have legalized a blending of milk and butterfat, but he claimed that he had become involved because Commissioner Amster requested that he do so. Brown believed that changing the standards might result in lower prices without endangering public health. He confirmed that he had attended numerous professional meetings with the encouragement of his superiors. He categorically denied the allegation that he had used his office hours and staff for personal work. Along with responses to all known charges against him, the brief contained numerous letters endorsing his work.[53]

The hearing ended with Copeland expressing admiration for

the professional accomplishments of Brown, a hint that the board was about to reinstate him. Another month dragged on, however, without any word as to his fate. Finally, on 10 August, the board announced its decision that the director was to be reinstated and suggested that the blame for his poor administrative record may have rested with his former superiors. They reprimanded him for the methods that he had used in the administration of his bureau, distorting much of the material that he had offered as a defense, and gave instructions for his future conduct. Brown soon responded to the public statement of the board: "There are so many inaccuracies, and some of the conclusions drawn seem to me so much without adequate foundation, that I should not feel that I were just to myself, if I did not enter a respectful rejoinder to it, and I therefore request leave to file this reply." He added that "due regard for disciplinary requirements" prevented him from making a statement to the press. Among the inaccuracies that he recognized was the contention that his failure to draft standards had resulted in the loss of court suits. The cases cited by the board to support its opinion had been initiated prior to his appointment. He also denied having said that adulterated food had little effect on public health, a claim made by the board.[54]

During the hot summer months, interest in the war between the politicians and the health experts lagged. When Brown was reinstated, the press in general took little note of the event. The *American* seemed pleased with the decision, especially because of the blame assigned to former commissioners of health for Brown's alleged dereliction of duty, but the *Tribune* expressed emphatically the opinion of most of the newspapers: "The last chapter in the Hylan fiasco which started with the mayor's drive on the Health Department last spring was closed yesterday, when Dr. Lucius Polk Brown, was reinstated unanimously by the Board of Health."[55]

Brown himself had realized that he was merely a pawn in a power play. When Alice Lakey, president of the Village Improvement Association, had written him a flowery premature congratulatory letter just after the hearing, the director revealed that he had no illusions about the situation. Miss Lakey gushingly penned the following message: "It is interesting to note how the aspect of the whole affair has altered since it became apparent that you were a man of National reputation, with hosts of important men standing ready to vouch for you. The miserable clique that fought you did not know that they were putting their necks in jeopardy." Brown replied: "Most people seem to have already made up their minds in the matter, so that the action the Board may take will have little effect on the situation in one way—but I trust they will have intelligence enough to find a good way out of it for both of us."[56]

The Board of Health did find "a good way out of it" for Brown and themselves. They failed to disavow charges that Copeland had made against him, but they absolved the director of most of the responsibility by placing the blame for his actions on former commissioners—Goldwater, Emerson, and Amster. Copeland had represented the interests of Tammany well. He had stepped into the job of commissioner after the machine was under heavy attack because of the blundering of Hylan and had saved Smith, Murphy, and others from further embarrassment. He received his reward when Smith balked on a deal made between Murphy and McCooey to back Hearst for the United States Senate in 1922. Murphy may not have been particularly interested in a Hearst candidacy, but outwardly he maintained a neutral position rather than split his party. Eventually, Hearst, in the face of opposition from Smith, agreed to step down if he could name the candidate—Dr. Royal S. Copeland. Smith concurred, and he and Copeland went on to victory in the fall. Copeland emerged from the struggle of 1918 as a master politician. He had not alienated Tammany, Hearst, or Hylan, the inept sidekick of the newspaperman.[57]

Copeland came out of the struggle in better condition than anyone else. By autumn 1918 the turmoil had subsided, and opponents looked over the field of battle and counted their casualties. Reformers and the experts at the Department of Health had won the battle of the directorships—the bureaus survived—but they had lost the war. The Department of Health had been ravaged by politics. Indeed, so affected was it by the fury of the fight, that the *Annual Report* of 1917 did not appear in print until August of the following year—and this breakdown was among a group of experts who excelled in writing reports.

The Mitchelites had their reforms devastated before their very eyes. The experts, through their resignations, and the reformers, through their division into splinter groups supporting this bureau or that, had played into the hands of politicians. Furthermore, the results of their failure to secure civil-service status for the post of commissioner became evident. It was through that office that the professional politicians played havoc with the department. The reformers had built a "model" organization, but they had been unable to complete the protective wall around it. Worst of all for them, they realized their folly. A decade after Tammany had tried to purge the New York City Department of Health, Charles-Edward A. Winslow, who had served as a harbinger of danger in 1918, aptly described the tragedy: "Ten years ago it was beyond question that New York City had the best municipal health department in the world. In 1918 came a change, and for the first time in thirty years the blight of political influence fell upon the splendid social machinery."[58]

Reformers and professional scientists had bowed to the show of force by professional politicians. Government, in New York City at least, still remained almost exclusively in the domain of politicians, primarily because of the myopia of reformers. Nonetheless, inroads had been made in government that caused the politicians a great deal of difficulty. The Brown hearing had demonstrated the problem of removing a competent public servant protected by civil-service regulations if he chose to fight rather than resign.

The two opposing power blocs had struggled for control of health administration. In the long run, neither side gained much. The bureaus, significantly weakened, survived as vestiges of reform ascendancy. Nonetheless, the old efficiency had been destroyed, and politics permeated the department. In September, Copeland announced a plan that gave the boroughs a measure of influence in health matters. He named Frank J. Monaghan as the new sanitary superintendent, and he appointed five assistants at the borough level. The directors of the bureaus were forced to confer with the sanitary superintendent on all controversial matters; the commissioner served as final arbiter. The Citizens Union accepted this move as a symbolic victory. They tended to see preservation of the bureaus as an end in itself. This strategy, however, rendered the directors nothing more than figureheads. Permitting politics to infiltrate, the plan was thus incorporated into the general health administration. Hylan, with no obvious embarrassment, campaigned in later years on the basis of administrative competence and health achievements. His propagandists proclaimed, "A is for Administration—the best New York has ever had," and "H is for Health and Hospitals."[59]

The professional politicians also took some losses. Copeland served them as a willing tool, but serving willingly did not necessarily mean serving well. He held the office of commissioner of health until he was elected to the Senate. When he resigned, Frank Monaghan assumed the post—a promotion made easier by his previous elevation to the office of deputy commissioner. As head of the Department of Health, Monaghan allowed corruption and graft to envelop the establishment. The decline was brought home to New Yorkers when James J. Walker defeated Hylan in the Democratic primary of 1925 and became mayor. During Walker's administration, the new commissioner of health, Louis I. Harris, the former director of the Bureau of Preventable Diseases, uncovered the profusion of corruption that Monaghan had fostered, an abundance of which permeated the Bureau of Food and Drugs.[60]

Revelations tended to confirm what some citizens had always thought about politicians—that they were corrupt and not to be trusted but that they occasionally offered a welcome relief as replacements for the "highbrows." The surviving reformers, scientific experts, and Mitchelites were avenged by the evidence that was unearthed by Harris and his associates. The Department of Health had become a tool of politicians, and as such, it was an instrument of patronage and a ready-made source of corrupt profit—just as the experts and reformers had warned when they stood like shivering Cassandras before the Hylan onslaught of 1918.

The power blocs survived the war intact, but a number of individuals fell by the wayside. James E. MacBride, the obnoxious chairman of the Civil Service Commission, stepped down on 7 June under pressure to do so from his own camp because of the wrath that he had caused to be heaped upon them. Two health commissioners, Haven Emerson and J. Lewis Amster, did not survive the Hylan purge. Former commissioner S. S. Goldwater, a holdover from the Mitchel administration, resigned his seat on the Medical Advisory

Board. Directors, it seemed, were also expendable. Dr. Charles F. Bolduan resigned from the Bureau of Public Health Education in May. Dr. F. B. Krause, sanitary superintendent, lasted until August. The final bureau to come under siege during this war was Preventable Diseases, headed by Harris. In January 1919, Copeland set out to remove the Division of Industrial Hygiene from his direction. Although reformers had suffered heavy casualties, they, along with labor and civic leaders, rose up in such fury that the commissioner let the matter drop. Lucius Polk Brown held the unique distinction of being the only director to be vindicated of charges leveled against him by the Hylan administration.[61]

Brown had nothing to lose from a public investigation; a private inquiry he feared. He chose to fight Hylan and Copeland through the press. He met the plot to remove him head-on and won. Successfully defending his honor, he had no delusions about the implications. The character of the individual expert had been subverted when the directors became the pawns in a power play. Brown and the others were held up to public ridicule, demoralized, and deprived of any real authority. They could no longer take pride in their association with the New York City Department of Health. Brown was a victim of the war on experts. Too stubborn to resign, he looked to the military for a way out.

8—The Exit of a Scientist: From Public Service to Private Citizenship, 1918-35

The New York health controversy of 1918 altered the life of Lucius Polk Brown. Although it did not lessen his interest in service to his country or his concern for public health, it diminished his enthusiasm for his career as a food and drug control official. A short stint with the military and a brief, unsuccessful return to New York City represented his only significant gestures toward public service. From 1918 until his death in 1935, Brown expressed his opinions, for the most part, as a private citizen. During this period he occupied himself with farming and enjoyed the tranquility of his family. Occasionally, however, the old flashes of reformism and liberalism surfaced, leading him to speak out on various issues.

The pure food and drug movement lost some of its momentum during the 1920s. At the federal level, officials struggled to keep up the fight, armed with the old law of 1906, which had long failed to cope with changing conditions.[1] In Tennessee and New York City the effort languished. Brown lived to witness the first battles over proposed food, drug, and cosmetic legislation during the New Deal, a measure sponsored by his old adversary, Senator Royal S. Copeland. This was more than a decade away from the immediate problem he faced in 1918—how to make a graceful exit from an unpleasant situation. The war, for him, served as a timely excuse.

World War I was a milestone of the Progressive era. Its effect on individuals and particular groups of reformers, however, varied.

Historians have found the impact of the war to be almost as perplexing and fascinating as Progressivism itself. Vernon L. Parrington rendered the following epitaph: "Then the war intervened and the green fields shriveled in an afternoon. With the cynicism that came with post-war days the democratic liberalism of 1917 was thrown away like an empty whiskey-flask." Allen F. Davis perceived of the war as a boost for social workers who participated in one of the many phases of Progressivism. "The war," according to him, "came as a great shock to the social workers; at first it seemed to spell the end of social reform. Yet gradually, to their own surprise, many of them came to view the war, despite its horror and its danger, as a stimulus to their promotion of social justice in America." Davis also pointed out that the war seemed to put an end to dissension among social workers and allowed them to delude "themselves into thinking that the social experiments and social action of the war years would lead to even greater accomplishments in the reconstruction years ahead."[2]

Instead of killing reformism or promoting it, however, the war provided an excuse for some liberals to divorce themselves from crusades that had already lost momentum. Historians since the 1950s have found it fashionable to search for class origins and economic motivations of the Progressives, but in their scholarly arguments, they have not cast aside the fervent patriotism and nationalism that characterized this generation of liberals.[3] Parrington aptly described them as "a school dedicated to the ideals of the Enlightenment and bent on carrying through the unfulfilled program of democracy."[4] When the United States became involved in the European war, some Progressives found that their patriotism permitted them to exit gracefully from the reform scene. This is not to imply that their patriotism was a ruse, but it did prove a useful attribute for some disillusioned domestic crusaders.

From the moment that the Progressives injected their ideas into the American political cauldron at the local level, they fought continuous battles in a philosophical and ideological conflict that eventually spread from the cities and states through the nation. By 1917, when the United States entered a foreign war, the steam had gone out of some of the reform efforts. The same patriotism that had helped to spur internal reform allowed some Progressives to retreat honorably from their collapsing skirmish lines. The First World War provided such men as Lucius Polk Brown and John Purroy Mitchel, his one-time administrative superior, a graceful exit. When duty called, no patriotic American could refuse its summons.

Essentially these were the sentiments that Brown expressed when he requested a leave of absence from his position in New York City. He wrote to Copeland:

> I have been offered a commission as Captain in the Foods and Nutrition Division of the Sanitary Corps, Surgeon General's Office, United States Army. You are doubtless informed fully as to the important functions of this division in the sustenance of the army. I am reliably informed that the need for men is great and I know that the supply of men qualified for this work is not very large. Under these circumstances I must regard this request as a call to serve and I could not with self-respect disregard it. I, therefore, apply for a leave of absence without pay for the term of the war.[5]

After Hylan launched his war on experts, Brown had begun looking for new employment. Before his fate at the Department of Health had been decided, he considered two alternatives, private business and military service. On 20 July 1918, Major John F. Murlin of the Army Sanitary Corps asked if he were free to consider a commission with assignment to the Division of Food and Nutrition. Brown replied that before he could give Murlin a definite answer, he needed to settle two matters: first, an agreement with a private concern for work after the city controversy was resolved, and naturally, the second, his situation with the New York City Department of Health. The next day, Major Casper W. Miller of the Medical Reserve Corps, who had spoken with the director in New York, informed him that the surgeon general felt he could justifiably hold open a position for a man as experienced as Brown for at least a month.[6]

Soon after Brown had been reinstated, he notified the Office of the Surgeon General. Murlin congratulated Brown on his victory and urged him to settle his private affairs as soon as possible so that he could report to Camp Greenleaf, Fort Oglethorpe, Georgia. Brown needed no encouragement to sever his ties with the Department of

Health. Rumors were already circulating by the end of August that Commissioner Royal S. Copeland planned to change the administration of the department. His scheme called for depriving directors of most of their authority and transferring power to the sanitary superintendent and his borough assistants. By this time the director was most anxious to speed up his commission. As he told Major Murlin:

> Since I wrote you, certain things have come to my knowledge which, metaphorically speaking, make the prognosis, so far as the Health Department is concerned, very uncertain, not only for me but for other Directors. It therefore appears that it is desirable for me to sever my connection with that body as early as is decent. I therefore hope that I can get to you some time during the month of September. Obviously, however, I do not wish to leave them until the matter of my connection with your Division is definitely settled, so that I am doing all I can to help you push it.[7]

On 30 September, Copeland granted Brown a formal leave of absence. A New York newspaper carried a note on the financial sacrifice involved. As captain in the Sanitary Corps, he would receive only $2,400 a year. This salary, less than half that of the director, possessed the security that the other one lacked. Although the army provided Brown with the way out of a difficult situation, military service, nonetheless, was a family tradition; and the captain's son, Marine Lieutenant Campbell Brown, a career man, had sailed for France during the summer with the famous Thirteenth Regiment, commanded by Colonel Smedley D. Butler. When Brown accepted the commission, he arranged for his wife and three daughters to return to Tennessee.[8]

Brown belonged to the first generation of American health experts, exclusive of physicians, to make a significant contribution in a military conflict. The United States Army in World War I, to a greater extent than any American army before it, had the knowledge and ability to maintain high health standards. Whereas health and sanitation concerns had been something of a fad in the Spanish-American War, they became matters for paramount consideration twenty years later. This alteration can be attributed to the "new" public health movement that transpired in the United States after the turn of the twentieth century.[9]

By the end of the Progressive era, health reformers assumed responsibility for the protection of the individual from dangers beyond his control. They believed that by safeguarding the individual, society, as a whole, stood to reap the benefits. Into a realm that previously had been the exclusive domain of physicians, there now ventured social workers, nurses, muckrakers, concerned citizens, and scientists. With so many types of people participating in the effort, the perspective on health became much broader during the Progressive period. No longer was public health viewed as the mere absence of disease. On 24 October 1916, in a paper presented to the American Public Health Association, W. C. Rucker, assistant surgeon general of the United States Public Health Service, pointed to the need for broad vision. He called for a public health policy embracing "the political economy of disease, and far reaching as human nature, since after all, human nature is the groundwork from which arises the public health." Four years later, Charles-Edward A. Winslow, a professor of public health at the Yale School of Medicine, defined the "new" public health. He stressed "the science and the art of preventing disease, prolonging life, and promoting physical health and efficiency through organized community efforts."[10]

This new spirit in America inspired the following comment in a publication prepared by the Surgeon General's Office during World War I:

> Any account of advances made in military sanitation in our Army during the period between the Spanish-American War and the World War would be very incomplete if no reference were made to the development of the sanitary conscience of the Army in the meantime. With the American public as a whole, from which, of course, our World War Army came— and this also doubtless proved of considerable assistance in protecting the health of the troops—the same process had been going on.[11]

An interest in the purity of food as well as its nutritional value had been one of the many facets of the "new" public health movement. This aspect of civilian reform had its parallel in the military.

Origins of a food and nutrition sector can be traced to August 1917; officially, however, the Office of Food and Nutrition dated from 4 September. By 1918 it had found its way into the Surgeon General's Office, under the Division of Sanitation. It was also known as the Food and Nutrition Division of the Sanitary Corps, and after the armistice, it was called the Food and Nutrition Section of the Sanitation Division.[12]

On 20 September 1917 a conference had taken place at the headquarters of the United States Food Administration in Washington, D.C. Those in attendance—the surgeon general, the quartermaster general, a representative from the British army, the director of the federal food administration, and several experts—dealt with problems related to the food supply of the army. The most significant suggestion entertained by this group called for nutritional surveys of military camps. The secretary of war approved the idea on 16 October, and the adjutant general implemented it on 26 October.[13]

In addition to making sanitary surveys, the food and nutrition officers, who were being recruited as rapidly as possible, had responsibility for determining the nutritional value of food and the quality of the rations, for inspecting mess halls, and for halting food waste. The latter problem required careful attention because the army came under harsh censure from sacrificing civilians throughout the country when even a trace of wastefulness could be found. Angry citizens from the Pacific Coast to the piney woods of Georgia fired off a barrage of letters to newspaper editors and public officials. Some complained that the portions served were so large that the soldiers left food on their plates, which had to be thrown away. Others pointed out that cooks always prepared the same amounts, even when the enlisted men had weekend passes. Officers were scorned for their customary extravagances. An editorial from the *Hamilton County* (Georgia) *Herald*, criticizing waste at Fort Oglethorpe, Georgia, echoed sentiments similar to those elsewhere in the country:

> A Negro cook for one of the companies sat upon the street car on Saturday night last. He told his fellow negro passengers a story about how much was thrown out that night at supper.
> He stated that he had orders to prepare supper for 170

men in the mess he cooked for. When supper came but eight sat down to eat it. Potatoes enough, wheat bread enough, salmon croquettes enough, white beans and an entire box of prunes which had been cooked together with pastry was all THROWN INTO THE SLOP PAILS.[14]

Such accusations had some validity. Suffice it to say that the food administration and the army made an effort to cope with these criticisms.

At first the staff of the Food and Nutrition Division came from the faculties of medical schools, university laboratories, agricultural experiment stations, and state and municipal food control authorities. These individuals required only a brief course of training in army procedure, in the conduct of nutritional surveys, and in the inspection of large quantities of food. Officers commissioned in the division reported directly to Washington, D.C., where they were subjected to a series of lectures and practical demonstrations. The Bureau of Chemistry and food officials from the District of Columbia cooperated with the army in this venture. Later, on 7 March 1918, a special course for nutrition officers was established at Camp Greenleaf. Instruction there suffered from one major handicap, the lack of laboratory facilities.[15]

Reports indicated that the Food and Drug Division attained a strength of 116 men by the end of the war, including 1 lieutenant colonel, 8 majors, 35 captains, 36 first lieutenants, and 36 second lieutenants. As rapidly as possible, these men were sent to the training camps. When officers became available, each base of more than 10,000 men received a designated expert, sometimes assisted by enlisted personnel. Even before it became known that nutrition officers were being readied for service, commanders of training camps recognized the need for their expertise and requested that such men be assigned to their posts. After February 1918, even the American Expeditionary Forces employed the services of the division—36 specialists boarded ships for Europe during 1918, 6 in March, 20 in June and July, and 10 in November.[16]

Shortly after the armistice the army began discharging such personnel, but some officers remained on duty at debarkation stations. Brown was in training at Camp Greenleaf when the fighting ceased, and he spent the duration of his service inside the country. After his initial indoctrination, he received orders for Camp Bowie, Texas. He remained in Texas from December 1918 to April 1919, spent a short period at Post Field Aviation Camp, Fort Sill, Oklahoma, and Ellington Field at Houston, Texas, whereupon he was transferred to the debarkation point at Hoboken. He stayed in New Jersey until he was discharged on 19 July 1919. Even then, his connection with the military remained in effect until he resigned his commisson as captain in the Officers' Reserve Corps in 1924.[17]

When Brown had left New York for Camp Greenleaf, he turned in his badge as "Director of Bureau" and probably had no intention of returning to his job. After his discharge from active duty, however, he decided to avail himself of the salary until he could find more satisfying employment. When he again took up his duties as director in late July, he and Commissioner Copeland began an exchange of argumentative notes on subjects ranging from such major problems as the enforcement hierarchy to such petty ones as the location of offices. The root of their differences centered on the decentralization of the Bureau of Food and Drugs. The authority that had once rested with the directors had been dissipated throughout the boroughs among the assistant sanitary superintendents. Blame for failures to enforce the sanitary code effectively could still be thrust on men who headed the bureaus. Brown resented being placed in such a predicament, but he received no sympathy from the commissioner.

When the director complained that his *drug division* had been weakened, Copeland responded: "I am sorry that there has to creep into so many of your official communications some plaintive note relative to 'what is left' of your Bureau. It seems to be very difficult for you to understand that nothing has been taken from your Bureau, and the sooner you appreciate this fact, the more comfortably you will pursue your ordinary duties."[18] He elaborated on this theme in another communication written on the same day: "I trust I have made clear to you in unmistakable language, that you have the responsibility of your Bureau, and that you have back of you the full authority of the Commissioner of Health to enforce every reasonable regulation. The summer season is over now, vacations must be forgotten, and every Director is expected to functionate to the benefit of society." The commissioner added that Brown should forget "all gossip" and confine himself "to conditions as they actually exist."[19]

Along with their disagreements over decentralization of authority, Brown and Copeland also clashed over changes in personnel. In July 1919, Copeland had designated Ole Salthe, formerly assistant director of the Bureau of Food and Drugs, the supervising chief food inspector and head of the Division of General Reference and had assigned him to duty in his own office. When Brown questioned the legitimacy of such a move under Salthe's civil-service title and when Brown balked at signing the payroll roster, Copeland lashed out: "It is very plain to me that Mr. Salthe is serving the Department efficiently and successfully and is working within his civil service title." Copeland had a much better relationship with Salthe than with Brown. After he went to the Senate, Salthe became his chief legislative assistant.[20]

Contrary to assurances by Copeland, Brown no longer had authority to direct his bureau. The commissioner repeatedly reminded the director of his power, for the written record, but held up communications from the borough chiefs concerning hearings on matters for which Brown was responsible. Obviously such a situation could not long endure. Beginning in October, Brown requested leaves of absence without pay, which kept him away from the department through December 1920.[21]

The disputes between Copeland and Brown deprived the Department of Health of valuable expertise that could have been put to good use in the drug-addiction program implemented in New York City during 1919. It shared the major attributes of the plan that Brown had developed in Tennessee. Beginning on 7 July, under the Public Health Law of New York State, every person in New York City who was addicted to cocaine or its derivatives had to register with an agent of the State Department of Narcotic Drug Control before he could secure a prescription for such drugs. Walter R. Herrick, commissioner of the Department of Narcotic Control, designated the commissioner of the municipal Department of Health as the official agent. Copeland estimated that the city might have as many as 200,000 addicts. During 1919, however, only 6,579 addicts registered—5,047 males and 1,532 females. The peak age period for both sexes was 21 to 30. Whites accounted for 5,778 of the total;

blacks, 796; and Orientals, 5. New York City authorities also experimented with a clinical approach to the treatment of heroin addicts, but they decided by 1920 to close the treatment service and to institutionalize the serious cases.[22]

With Brown out of the city during most of 1920, Copeland and the legal authorities there seemed to take delight in ordering him to appear for trials. The matter of corruption in the bureau, which had arisen in 1918, carried over to 1920. Two inspectors, T. Spencer Duignan and Harold W. J. Keen, had been indicted by a grand jury on 2 May 1918. Their cases remained before the court until 1920, and Brown was subpoenaed repeatedly. They both went free when Judge Rosalsky dismissed the indictment against Duignan on 15 March and found Keen not guilty on the same day.[23]

The ridiculous status of Brown with the Department of Health did neither him nor the board any credit. Apparently the director chose to maintain his tenuous relationship out of sheer obstinacy, and the commissioner had no valid excuse for denying him a leave of absence. Finally, after a year of this on-again, off-again employment, Brown submitted his resignation on 27 December 1920, effective 31 December.[24]

The experience of Brown as a food and drug control official had been a disillusioning one. When he had left Tennessee, he had the satisfaction of knowing that he had established a viable department which had public support. When he left New York City, he had the distinct impression that the authority of his bureau had been undermined. Even worse, during his absence from his native state, the Tennessee department had declined under the supervision of a man with less ability, being reduced principally to the duty of enforcing state liquor laws and serving as a mouthpiece for the federal food administration. When Harry L. Eskew, his successor, resigned as commissioner, Governor A. H. Roberts appointed George Draper to the post. Draper had worked with the department when Brown was the commissioner but had not impressed his superior. When the announcement was made, Brown, who may have had hopes of returning to that office in Tennessee, denounced the appointment because Draper was a pharmacist, not "a chemist of established reputation and ability," as the law specified he should be.[25]

Worse still, the federal food and drug law had proved to be a disappointment. In 1906, when it was passed, lobbyists for the bill had generally considered it to be no more than a foundation, although later, Harvey W. Wiley seemed to view it as a perfect piece of legislation. Even Brown, as president of the Association of American Dairy, Food and Drug Officials during 1912, took a dim view of enforcement under the Pure Food and Drug Act of 1906. "It must be said that the United States courts," he noted, "have succeeded in taking a large proportion of the teeth out of the Federal food and drugs act of June 30, 1906." On the other hand, at that time, he remained optimistic about the cooperation between states and municipalities. In 1914 some reformers went so far as to call the federal law a farce and nothing more than an honest-label law. By the 1920s federal officials were beset with problems that could not be solved by execution of the old law.[26]

Several prominent first-generation food and drug experts had resigned their positions and receded into the background of American life by the 1920s. Harvey W. Wiley, Robert M. Allen, and Lucius Polk Brown represented prime examples. The political fights, the lost arguments, and their own ambition had drained them of the old stamina. The decisions of these individuals and other reformers to resign from public offices that they had helped to create left the country with a legacy of expanding bureaucracies, headed by people who were often placed in high positions at the whim of politicians. Therefore, one of the most undesirable by-products of Progressivism was that bureaucracies remained which could be manipulated by politicians and managed by their inept and incompetent appointees. Designed to implement reforms, these structures could also provide a secure nest for patronage seekers. This danger manifested itself particularly in Tennessee during the tenure of Brown's successor. Eskew, who was not legally qualified for the position, failed to maintain the integrity of the department and failed to ensure its detachment from the enforcement of prohibition laws. Furthermore, Progressive laws, including the federal pure food and drug act, were, out of political necessity, short-term compromise measures; reformers had expected to strengthen them in the future. With the resignation of those who had crusaded for the initial legislation, the further weakening of the laws by judicial decisions, and the ensuing antiregulatory attitude of the 1920s, even the efforts of capable administrators were thwarted.

When Brown resigned from the directorship in New York City, he returned to his farm at Brook Hill, near Franklin, Tennessee; acted as custodian of some cotton land that his family owned in Bolivar County, Mississippi; and looked for another salaried job. Between 1920 and 1923 he became a promotion agent of the Merrell-Soule Company of Syracuse, New York. Early in the century, Merrell-Soule had purchased a patent from Robert Stauf of Posen, Germany, for dessicating blood and milk, and in 1905 the company perfected the patent. During 1917, Brown had considered the idea an interesting one and had written articles on the advantages of dehydration as a method for preserving food. While he was with this firm, he helped to develop a dried-milk product called Klim, *milk* spelled backwards. The substance to be reconstituted had to be mixed with water and beaten vigorously. As a result of this venture, the Brown family had quantities of Klim on hand.[27]

When Brown tired of this enterprise, he again returned to farming. His mother had died, and he and his brother Percy, the only surviving children, had inherited Ewell Farm. They sold the estate, but the purchaser was unable to pay for it. The brothers repossessed the farm and sold it at auction, whereupon Lucius bought tracts totaling more than two hundred acres. He moved his family in November 1923 to the land where his relatives had lived even prior to the Civil War.[28]

Before Brown committed himself entirely to the agrarian life, he made one last effort to find a place for himself in the business world. This resulted in his employment as administrator general of the American Dairy Products Company in Havana, Cuba, for approximately a year and a half. This connection ended, however, when his superiors urged him to bribe health officials in Cuba. In righteous indignation he declared that "he had never taken a bribe and he never expected to give one," whereupon he made a swift departure for the mainland and rejoined his family in Tennessee.[29]

Fifty-eight years old in 1925, Brown devoted the last ten years of his life to his farm and his family. Public service and business ventures, by this time, held few if any attractions for him. Since 1908 his life had been a full one, with many activities that sometimes separated him from his children. Even during his many absences, however, he had been a loving father who took time to write personal tender notes to each of his children. He found the leisure to accompany them on long conversational walks and extended camping trips. According to one of his daughters, Brown seemed "a rather severe and serious man" but one who had "a good sense of humor." She had a great respect for his intelligence and recalled that he took time to answer questions about "nature, religion, eternity, almost anything you wanted to talk about."[30]

Father to three lively girls, husband to an intelligent woman, and son of a strong-willed southern lady, Brown favored political and economic opportunities for females. He had supported female suffrage long before it was a reality, and he advocated professional and vocational training for young women. At a time when most of his blue-blood relatives thought finishing schools more suitable for girls than four-year colleges, he encouraged his daughters to continue their education. All three earned degrees from the University of Tennessee during the late 1920s. Impatient with southerners who boasted of their ancestry, he advised his children: "Don't be a professional descendant; be an ancestor yourself."[31]

A devoted family man, Brown nonetheless was too complex a personality to refuse an invitation to a White House Conference on Child Health and Protection that was called by President Herbert Hoover in 1929. Such conclaves as this temporarily brought the old liberals back into the limelight. When specialists gathered in Washington to share their ideas, Brown discussed the methods for controlling animal diseases that are transmitted to humans through milk, especially tuberculosis and undulant fever. He did not attend all the sessions, but his name appeared on a list of participants during July 1930, along with such well-known figures as Grace and Edith Abbott, S. Josephine Baker, Sophonisba Breckinridge, Ernest W. Burgess, Frances Perkins, Lawrence Veiller, Lillian Wald, Harvey Zorbaugh, and Haven Emerson. Seeing his former associates from New York—Wald, Emerson, and Baker—probably led Brown to reflect on the Hylan disaster, which still rested uneasily on his mind.[32]

The New York health controversy had proved a godsend for Royal S. Copeland. As commissioner of health, Copeland gained the respect of the Tammany organization and used that position as a stepping stone to the United States Senate. A compromise candidate, he went to Washington in 1923 and held office until his death in 1938. Perhaps, he even entertained ideas of winning the Democratic nomination for the presidency in 1932. At any rate, he hardened toward the actual nominee, and on inauguration day, his entire staff remained on the job. In 1933, Senator Copeland sponsored a new food, drug, and cosmetics bill. All the old arguments reappeared as reformers and their opponents girded themselves for a fight. By 1934 the Copeland measure had been weakened considerably. Oswald Garrison Villard, of the liberal *Nation*, revealed that the opposition was putting pressure on newspaper editors, columnists, and cartoonists to help defeat the bill, and he questioned Copeland's support of the altered proposal. Villard warned:

> As a physician sincerely interested in protecting the public health and the public pocket-book, Senator Copeland—who has publicly approved the emasculated bill—must know that this bill is badly damaged. As a politician, he should be informed that if he fails to denounce the emasculation of his bill on the floor of the Senate, he will hear from his constituency on next election day. And he had better not try appealing to them on radio time sponsored by patent-medicine manufacturers.[33]

Brown, meanwhile, followed the Copeland bill with considerable interest. He wrote to Villard after the editorial appeared, apparently denouncing the senator, for Villard expressed interest in securing copies of correspondence between Brown and Copeland. James Rorty of Wesport, Connecticut, a friend of Villard's and a contributor to the *Nation*, was at that time doing research for a book on Copeland. Brown put together a file on the New York controversy and offered it to Rorty. Brown obviously desired to have his record cleared, but he expressed himself mildly when he wrote to Villard: "Dr. Copeland's tinkering with the Health Department I believe set back its development very materially, and destroyed much good already accomplished." In a letter to Rorty, Brown minced no words:

All circumstances connected with Copeland's assumption of the Health post in New York indicated a set attack by the patent medicine crowd, since they centered their fire on Bolduan, publicity director, and myself—who joined the N.Y. force as much for the apparent opportunity to enforce the New York ordinances as for any other single reason. Well, I gave 'em all the H— I could while I was there and before I went there, and I'm proud of it. Incidentally, I must take my hat off to Copeland as the slickest bird in the game.[34]

While memories of the New York controversy continued to haunt Brown, he also had financial difficulties. During the agricultural depression of the 1920s he had overextended his farming operations, taking out mortgages to buy more equipment and new foundation stock. His tendency to overestimate his business abilities may have stemmed from the days of his youth, when Ewell Farm had been run on a more lavish scale. His economic situation was easing, however, after Franklin D. Roosevelt became president and Congress began to grind out relief measures for farmers.[35]

Whatever advantages Brown enjoyed from the relief efforts of the New Deal, he was neither swept up in the Roosevelt hysteria nor particularly enamored with the Democratic party. He read attentively the proposal of Mark Granite for a United Liberal party, and he gave Granite the following assessment of the political mood of the South: "As to the matter of the Liberal Party, I fear that at present in the South, there is, except locally, no Democratic nor Republican Party— it's a Roosevelt Party." "Hell and high water," he observed, "have no terrors for these folks if only Roosevelt will lead them."[36]

Politics still intrigued Brown, pure food and drugs interested him, and anxieties over old reform campaigns haunted him. He would not live to see the end of Roosevelt's first term or the eventual passage of the Copeland bill in 1938. His last years were filled with serious health problems, including chronic indigestion, mental depression, and coronary ailments. On 4 April 1935, Brown, sixty-eight years old, died of a heart attack, which had occurred the day before. At the time of the seizure, he was working on a series of articles for the *Columbia Herald*, a local newspaper.[37]

The period from 1918 to 1935 had been anticlimactic for Brown when compared to his other adult years. Smarting from the humiliation that he had suffered in 1918 and genuinely wanting to serve his country, he had turned to the military as the way out of a deplorable situation. His brief return to New York City only confirmed what he had feared. The bureaus over which scientific experts had once proudly presided had been riddled by petty politics and had been deprived of authority. Only hollow structures remained to be filled by patronage seekers. As an honorable man, he could not accept the changes that he observed. Brown turned from public service to private business and agriculture. Farming had always been a pleasant sideline for him; the country, a refuge from the tempestuousness of the offices he had held. As a full-time venture it offered no satisfactory outlet for the civic obligations that he felt. The reunion of reformers that Herbert Hoover summoned at the end of the 1920s gave him and other old first-generation liberals of the twentieth century a chance to surface before they were supplanted by a new vintage—in the 1930s.

9—Lucius Polk Brown
and Progressive Food and Drug Control:
Historical Perspectives

Fated for a public career during those tempestuous decades when the United States swayed under the weight of modern social forces and then carried them over into the twentieth century, Lucius Polk Brown was both a product of his times and a molder of them. A southerner, Brown divested himself of the trappings of an old regionalism and donned the cloak of nationalism; cast in the agricultural-experiment-station pattern, he perceived of problems that transcended rural America; a professional chemist, he sought a career in public service; and a social reformer, he operated in bureaucratic structures. He was a member of a "new middle class," one of many socially conscious, dedicated professionals who sought order out of chaos through efficiency, continuity, rationality, and smooth-running governmental bureaucracies.

Brown the reformer operated in the microcosmic domain of pure food and drug control. He joined other professionals to ferret out adulterated and misbranded products, seek honest labeling, and determine standards of purity. His sphere, however, was not a sterile one inhabited only by scientific experts. Politicians, businessmen, and other social reformers infringed on it and complicated his work. Health reformers, including food and drug experts, attempted to order their society through bureaucratic structures that were guarded by civil-service regulations and the powerful momentum of self-perpetuating establishments.

The career of Lucius Polk Brown in Progressive food and drug control at the state and municipal levels from 1908 to 1920 has afforded an opportunity for assessing this aspect of reform in a rural southern state and a huge northern metropolis. Such work carried with it some small successes, which in turn were diminished by the larger failures. The successes and the failures, too, developed within the framework of the bureaucracies that the crusaders created in order to implement change. The work of these particular Progressives must be measured within this context.

The relative ease with which Brown developed the Pure Food and Drug Department in Tennessee between 1908 and 1915, cultivated public opinion, and influenced state lawmakers could be attributed to the simplicity of the society in which he operated. By contrast, his inability to enlarge the Bureau of Food and Drugs in New York City, his limited influence in molding public opinion, and his vulnerability in the political fight of 1918 rested with the complexity of the environment in which he functioned. Whereas Tennessee had a rather homogeneous society, a one-party system for the most part, and an absence of well-defined power blocs, New York City encompassed a decidedly heterogeneous society; a permanent two-party system, which was often complicated by contesting Socialists and reformers; and highly developed power blocs that represented major interest groups, including professional politicians and scientists.

The levels of sophistication attained by northern and southern society influenced the possibilities for bureaucratic expansion and flexibility. In the South, very few restrictions were placed on Brown as a bureaucrat. Beginning with a one-man department in 1908, he increased the number of employees substantially to include two additional chemists, six inspectors, a stenographer, a porter, some temporary help, and local health officials who cooperated voluntarily. This rather amazing growth was made possible in a number of ways. First, the inspector managed, through valid arguments, to convince the general public, the press, and politicians that a definite need existed to enlarge his department in scope and usefulness. Second, he made his department a catchall for duties that did not logically fall into the domain of some other state agency. Although he complained about new responsibilities, including enforcement of a hotel law and weights and measures statutes in addition to the food and drug acts, acceptance of these duties allowed him to enlarge his department—a reality that he recognized.

Typical of bureaucrats in general, Brown never thought that his staff was adequate in size. In all likelihood, in this particular instance, his observations were valid. Every official report included renewed pleas for additional appropriations and more employees. Only with great reluctance did the state legislators loosen the purse strings. Nonetheless, in the great American tradition of political compromise, each time they met they found it possible to grant the inspector a small portion of what he wanted. Gradually, he built a viable department, one that was capable of sustaining and perpetuating itself when it came under fire in 1912.

The situation in New York City differed significantly. Brown was not "the big man" that he had been in Tennessee. He was only a cog in a machine, one that was already built and functioning. When he became a northern bureaucrat, he entered a more rigid system. In spite of his complaints that his bureau was not adequately staffed, he made no headway. Furthermore, he had less flexibility as an individual. In Tennessee he determined the needs for additional legislation, set standards, and formulated policy. He theoretically needed the approval of the Board of Health, but its members readily accepted his ideas. His retention of office rested directly with the governor. In the North he inherited a ready-made, fairly static bureau; his policy was already determined in large part by the municipal Sanitary Code; and he answered to the commissioner of health, a political appointee who depended on the favor of the mayor.

The quality of work conducted by the bureaucracies, North and South, hinged in part on the nature of the individual who directed them. Brown was an innovative person who was receptive to new ideas and willing to experiment. This helped to explain why he accepted the directorship in New York City. The job also seemed to be an improvement for him as a professional; he believed erroneously that the civil-service system in New York would free him from hassles over reappointment. The salary, too, was twice what he had received in Tennesssee, and the staff that he had at his disposal in the North dwarfed the one in the South. Interestingly enough, the inspectors in New York City received about the same pay as those in Tennessee, which hardly allowed them to keep pace with the cost of living in such a metropolis. Therefore, they were amazingly susceptible to bribery. This presented an administrative problem for the director. In Tennessee he maintained a firm paternalistic contol over his small force; in New York City the number of employees and the size of the city isolated his subordinates from his personal supervision.

The programs that Brown administered in Tennessee and New York City were shaped by his national vision. He attempted, in both environments, to correlate his work with other municipal, state, and federal officials. His affiliation with the national association of food and drug officials and similar professional organizations; his connections with such individuals as Harvey W. Wiley, Robert M. Allen, Willard D. Bigelow, and Carl Alsberg; and his acquaintance with social reformers operating in other spheres—all shaped his philosophy. His department in Tennessee profited from these relationships; such state politicians as Governors Patterson and Hooper did not resent a letter from Wiley, a suggestion from a federal official on weights and measures, or the professional affiliations of Brown. The Tennessee Pure Food and Drug Law of 1907 called for "a chemist of established reputation and ability," and the state legislature was reacting to congressional leadership when it passed the measure.

Acting contrary to the odium of States' rights, under which southern states labored after secession, Tennessee politicians, in the instance of health reform, were more responsive to federal directives than their New York counterparts. The New York City Department of Health enjoyed a unique kind of sovereignty because of state laws, and some machine politicians resented any activity that could be interpreted as state or federal interference. As a state official in Tennessee, Brown enjoyed a satisfactory working relationship with local and federal authorities; as a city official in New York, such opportunities were not always available. The tendency of New Yorkers to guard their autonomy in governmental matters, the size of the city, and the rivalry between boroughs complicated their relations with the state and federal government.

As for the practices that Brown sought to eliminate, the metropolitan New Yorkers had no monopoly on techniques for adulteration of food and drugs. Their country cousins and fellow urbanites in Tennessee were equally imaginative. The principal difference in the problems that Brown found in the two different environments was the greater magnitude caused by the situation in the tenement districts and the size and composition of the population. Furthermore, the work that had been conducted in the North prior to his employment there did not exceed in quality that of the same type in the South. When Brown assumed his duties in New York, he instituted the grading system, which he had established in Tennessee years earlier. His work in the South with drug addicts during 1914 and 1915 was strides ahead of that being done in New York City at the same time.

The success of Brown as a law-enforcement officer is difficult to evaluate. All the Progrssive campaigns were fraught with problems. The pure food and drug crusade was no exception. Real accomplishment rested on public acceptance and pressure from private citizens and interest groups. Initial concern for campaigns and raids against food and drug adulterators, on the part of citizens, usually lagged after the publicity accompanying them had subsided. Furthermore, Brown and others of his caliber were willing to accept the word of the dealers that they would conform; they prosecuted only as a last resort. Reformers, considering themselves men of honor, were too willing to acknowledge this trait in others. The campaign and the raid had influence only as long as the threat prevailed that dealers were under surveillance and could again be subjected to adverse publicity and prosecutions.

The short-term successes of the food and drug control experts in setting standards, prosecuting those who violated the laws, and winning public support represented manifestations of the larger problem that plagued the entire Progressive generation. Their greatest failure centered on the creation of hollow bureaucracies that were subject to political influence and incompetence. The microcosmic world of the pure food and drug workers illustrated this well. In Tennessee, society was not nearly so sophisticated as in New York City; the power blocs that Brown encountered in the North had no comparable counterparts in his home state. The only major opposition that he faced came in the latter part of 1911 and early 1912, when businessmen in Nashville and Davidson County mounted an unsuccessful campaign to prevent his reappointment. In this they did not enjoy the support of any political faction, in spite of the fact that they tried to cast the inspector, a Regular Democrat, as a political liability to Republican Governor Ben W. Hooper. The state executive, a Republican elected as a consequence of a fusion effort brought on by a split in the Democratic party over prohibition, refused to fall for their strategy. More of a gentlemanly reformer than a professional politician, he placed public service ahead of party loyalty.

The efforts of Brown in the South, therefore, benefited from the simplicity of his society. Because of the relative absence of interest groups and power elites, a positive program had greater chances for widespread acceptance. The unsuccessful effort of the businessmen of Nashville and Davidson County illustrate this point. Although this particular group opposed the inspector, they were unable to prevent his reappointment. The groups that supported Brown represented a grass-roots outpouring of support rather than a particular, highly organized power bloc motivated solely by a desire to keep him in office.

By way of contrast, two distinct, fairly well-matched groups—scientists and politicians—battled over the New York City Department of Health in 1918. The scientists had the support of a highly articulate hodgepodge of reformers, perhaps as much of a disadvantage as an advantage given their willingness to be content with the mere salvation of bureaus and given their efforts to save one bureau or another, not all of them collectively. As a consequence of the complexity of the environment, neither politicians nor scientists could obtain all of their objectives. Therefore, individuals fell by the wayside, and the efficiency of the Department of Health deteriorated. Even Lucius Polk Brown, who chose to fight rather than resign, became lost in the confusion around him.

The matter of professional loyalties influenced the whole episode of 1918. The truly professional politicians maintained allegiance to the machine. Even Boss Charles Francis Murphy and president of the Board of Aldermen Alfred E. Smith, who scorned such bungling and probably tempered the strategy of the mayor, put machine goals before service to the public, perhaps believing that they could serve the people best in this manner. As for the scientists, they, too, maintained their cohesion as professionals. Their respective societies rallied, and individuals rose to the occasion. Such experts as Royal S. Copeland and J. Lewis Amster were enigmas. Amster, for a while, accepted the leadership of Hylan but finally turned on him; Copeland served Hylan willingly.

The success that the New York City politicians had in undermining the Department of Health rested on the very nature of American politics at this point. When reformers brought pressure to bear, politicians were not strong enough to block the passage of legislation creating civil-service positions and jobs for idealists who were dedicated to constructive change, but neither were the Progressives strong enough to safeguard completely the bureaucracies that they created. They were not able to deprive politicians of their right to make appointments. This was true both in the rural South and in the urban North.

Although positions in the Pure Food and Drug Department in Tennessee were placed under civil-service regulations, the post of commissioner remained subject to appointment. The governor, therefore, had the power to influence and alter the choice of employees within the department because of the control that he exercised over the commissioner. After Brown left the state, Governor Rye ignored the law and appointed a man who was not qualified for the position; his successor, Governor Roberts, behaved likewise. In New York City, most vacancies in the Department of Health were filled by individuals who excelled on competitive examinations. The Board of Health, however, consisted of three members, two of whom were appointed by the mayor. Thus, the reform bureaucracies were open to infiltration by politicians.

Brown and reformers like him acted in good faith. They tried to make their world a better one. Attacking social abuses, they looked for ways to safeguard their achievements. Bureaucratic governmental machinery was the product of their rational minds. The first generation of twentieth-century American liberals, including food and drug reformers, failed to establish their ideal society because they could not break the influence of professional politicians. Not revolutionary, but sane and paradoxically conservative, they were victimized by aspects of the very institutions that they revered.

Bibliographical Note

The primary purpose of this book has been to provide a comparative study of scientific achievement and frustration at the state and municipal levels via the career of Lucius Polk Brown in Progressive food and drug control; research efforts have been directed toward unearthing materials having a bearing on the man as a scientist and as a Progressive reformer in Tennessee and New York City. Complete citations appear in the notes. The following, therefore, is a brief discussion of the sources that proved most useful.

MANUSCRIPTS

Because of the nature of this study, the papers of Lucius Polk Brown were of paramount importance. Unfortunately, these materials were not to be found in one large, indexed collection. The most valuable papers, those dealing with food and drug control in New York City and Tennessee, were in the possession of Susan Brown Lyon, Brown's oldest daughter, who resides at Murfreesboro, Tennessee. Because of his political tribulations in New York City, Brown himself had been concerned with the preservation of these records, believing that someday they might be of historical significance. When I first began to do research on this project in 1968, I sifted through those papers related to the Tennessee period and suggested that certain items be turned over to the Tennessee State Library and Archives, Nashville; Mrs. Lyon followed my suggestion. When I was completing this manuscript, the papers had not yet been indexed. Other Brown papers are in the possession of his daughter Lucia Brown Brownell, of Birmingham, Alabama. These include some newspaper clippings dealing with the New York work and a limited amount of correspondence for the period 1920 to 1935. A small Lucius Polk Brown Collection is housed at the James D. Hoskins Library, University of Tennessee, Knoxville. Most of these materials, however, relate to the agricultural activities of George Campbell Brown, Lucius Polk Brown's father, at Ewell Farm during the latter part of the nineteenth century.

Materials of an official nature, annual reports of the Tennessee Pure Food and Drug Inspector, correspondence related to the department, and papers dealing with Brown's employment as state chemist can be found in the Tennessee governors' papers, located at the Tennessee State Library and Archives. These include the papers of Governors James B. Frazier, Malcolm R. Patterson, Ben W. Hooper, and Tom C. Rye. Brown's articles and reports crop up in the *Biennial Report of the State Board of Health from January 1909 to January 1911*. Unfortunately, the reports were not published during four years of his administration in Tennessee. Also, his official message to a state agricultural convention appears in the *Biennial Report of the Department of Agriculture, 1909–1910*.

The massive collection of Harvey W. Wiley Papers, in the Library of Congress, Manuscripts Division, includes letters between Brown and Wiley and Wiley and other state food and drug officials. Coupled with the *Proceedings of the Association of State and National Food and Dairy Departments* for the annual conventions, they revealed the political activities of the national association of food and drug inspectors and the common problems of this rather tight-knit group.

A number of collections were consulted in an effort to come to terms with conditions as Brown found them in New York City. The materials located at the Haven Emerson Public Health Library were by far the most important to this study. The annual reports, bulletins, and newsletters provided a running account of the official activities of the Department of Health and the Bureau of Food and Drugs. Also, the archives there contained such invaluable resources as the *Collected Works of Haven Emerson*, Charles Bolduan's *Over a Century of Health Administration in New York City*, and departmental memoranda.

The politics affecting public health work in New York City receive lengthy treatment in this study. Those materials useful in understanding the prevailing climate were: the Citizens Union Papers, Lillian D. Wald Papers, and Edwin P. Kilroe Collection of Tammaniana, all housed at Columbia University's Butler Library. The scrapbooks in the Kilroe Collection were of inestimable value. Also, the public and private papers of mayors were enlightening. These include the public papers of Mayors John Purroy Mitchel and John F. Hylan, located at the Municipal Archives and Records Center in New York City, and the private papers of John Purroy Mitchel at the Library of Congress. The papers of Health Commissioner Royal S. Copeland, in the Michigan Historical Collections, University of Michigan, Ann Arbor, represented a large collection, very little of which dealt with Copeland's tenure as health commissioner. A few letters, however, shed considerable light on the controversy of 1918 and the views of those who opposed the health experts.

BIBLIOGRAPHICAL NOTE

INTERVIEWS

Because the papers of Lucius Polk Brown were not voluminous and because they represented only the highlights of his career, it is doubtful that this study could have been accomplished without the cooperation of Brown's children. I talked at length informally with Susan Brown Lyon and Colonel Campbell Brown on several different occasions. I recorded their formal statements. These talks, formal and informal, in 1968 and 1973, provided many insights that would otherwise have gone unnoticed.

Two other individuals whose recollections aided me considerably were: Thomas Ripley Bryant, retired director of extenson work at the Kentucky Agricultural Experiment Station in Lexington, and Mrs. Llewellyn H. King of Murfreesboro, Tennessee, one-time private secretary to Senator Royal S. Copeland. Mr. Bryant had been with the Agricultural Experiment Station in Kentucky in its early days and was familiar with the type of chemical analysis undertaken there; he had also been acquainted with a number of the first generation of food and drug control officials. Mrs. King was in poor physical condition, although she was quite alert mentally. I spoke with her by telephone concerning Copeland. She offered recollections about his personal habits and opinions.

GOVERNMENT PUBLICATIONS

Some government publications have been mentioned in connection with annual reports; others that were helpful to the study are mentioned below. The Tennessee House and Senate *Journals* provided information on the introduction of food and drug bills, their fate, the official vote, and how individual legislators stood on the issues. Debates were not included. The annual reports of the Tennessee Agricultural Experiment Station for 1889 and 1890 contained material on Brown's work as acting chemist. Annual reports of the United States Department of War for 1918 and 1919 and the United States Army, Surgeon General, study entitled *The Medical Department of the United States in the World War* included useful background information on the Food Division of the United States Army Sanitation Corps.

NEWSPAPERS

An intensive search through Tennessee and New York City newspapers proved quite rewarding in terms of facts yielded dealing with Brown's career from 1908 to 1915 in Tennessee and 1915 to 1920 in New York City. Newspapers are cited throughout the notes, but the *Nashville Tennessean*, the *Nashville Tennessean and American*, the *Nashville Banner*, the *New York Times*, and the *New York Herald* deserve particular recognition.

BIBLIOGRAPHICAL NOTE

BOOKS AND ARTICLES

The books and articles that influenced this work number in the hundreds, and those of direct bearing receive their much-deserved attention in the notes. A few books, however, must be singled out. These include: Oscar E. Anderson, Jr.,'s excellent study, *The Health of a Nation: Harvey W. Wiley and the Fight for Pure Food*; Paul E. Isaac's unsurpassed view of Tennessee politics in the late nineteenth and early twentieth centuries, *Prohibition and Politics: Turbulent Decades in Tennesse, 1885–1920*; Edwin R. Lewinson's equally useful account of New York politics in *John Purroy Mitchel: The Boy Mayor of New York*; Charles O. Jackson's analysis of the struggle for stronger federal controls, *Food and Drug Legislation in the New Deal*; Upton Sinclair's misbegotten revelation, *The Jungle*; and the old crusader's own story of his fights for food and drug control in *Harvey W. Wiley: An Autobiography*.

Notes

1. Not only has the topic of public health during the Progressive era received superficial treatment, but public health throughout American history has also been treated in a general manner by scholars. Expansive overviews of particular problems and studies based on nationally known figures characterize the pattern of this literature.

   Studies of an expansive nature include such works as John Duffy, *Epidemics in Colonial America* (Baton Rouge: Louisiana State University Press, 1953), *A History of Public Health in New York City, 1625–1866* (New York: Russell Sage Foundation, 1968), *A History of Public Health in New York City*, vol. 2: *1866–1966* (New York: Russell Sage Foundation, 1974); Charles E. Rosenberg, *The Cholera Years: The United States in 1832, 1849, and 1866* (Chicago: University of Chicago Press, 1962); John B. Blake, *Public Health in the Town of Boston, 1630–1822* (Cambridge, Mass.: Harvard University Press, 1959); Barbara Gutmann Rosenkrantz, *Public Health and the State: Changing Views in Massachusetts, 1842–1936* (Cambridge, Mass.: Harvard University Press, 1972); and David F. Musto, *The American Disease: Origins of Narcotic Control* (New Haven, Conn.: Yale University Press, 1973).

2. Studies that focus on specific aspects of public health within the context of Progressivism include Walter I. Trattner, *Homer Folks: Pioneer in Social Welfare* (New York: Columbia University Press, 1968); James H. Cassedy, *Charles V. Chapin and the Public Health Movement* (Cambridge, Mass.: Harvard University Press, 1962); Oscar E. Anderson, Jr., *The Health of a Nation: Harvey W. Wiley and the Fight for Pure Food* (Chicago: Published for the University of Cincinnati by the University of Chicago Press, 1958); and Stuart Galishoff, *Safeguarding the Public*

Health: Newark, 1895–1918 (Westport, Conn.: Greenwood Press, 1975). James Harvey Young has dealt with the subject of health quackery before and after federal regulation, and Charles O. Jackson has written an excellent account of the New Deal food and drug legislation. See Young, *The Toadstool Millionaires: A Social History of Patent Medicines in America before Federal Regulation* (Princeton. N.J.; Princeton University Press, 1961), and *The Medical Messiahs: A Social History of Health Quackery in Twentieth-Century America* (Princeton, N.J.: Princeton University Press, 1967); and Jackson, *Food and Drug Legislation in the New Deal* (Princeton, N.J.: Princeton University Press, 1970).

3. Everett C. Hughes, "Professions," in *The Professions in America*, ed. Kenneth S. Lynn and the editors of *Dædalus* (Boston, Mass.: Houghton Mifflin, 1965), pp. 1–14; Howard Mumford Jones, *The Age of Energy: Varieties of American Experience, 1865–1915* (New York: Viking Press, 1971), pp. 166–78; George H. Daniels, "The Process of Professionalization in American Science: The Emergent Period, 1820–1860," reprinted from *Isis* 58 (1967): 151–66, and "The Pure-Science Ideal and Democratic Culture," *Science* 156 (30 June 1967): 1699–1705.

4. Harold Zink, *City Bosses in the United States: A Study of Twenty Municipal Bosses* (Durham, N.C.: Duke University Press, 1930; reprint ed., New York: AMS Press, 1968), pp. 3–65, 128–63, 246–74, and 291–301; Nancy Joan Weiss, *Charles Francis Murphy, 1858–1924: Respectability and Responsibility in Tammany Politics* (Northampton, Mass.: Smith College, 1968); William D. Miller, *Mr. Crump of Memphis* (Baton Rouge: Louisiana State University Press, 1964); and Zane L. Miller, *Boss Cox's Cincinnati: Urban Politics in the Progressive Era* (New York: Oxford University Press, 1968).

5. Jones, *Age of Energy*, p. 336.

6. Herbert Croly, *The Promise of American Life* (New York: MacMillan, 1912), p. 118.

7. Quoted in David J. Rothman, *Politics and Power: The United States Senate, 1869–1901* (Cambridge, Mass.: Harvard University Press, 1966; New York: Atheneum Books, 1969), p. 111.

8. Lincoln Steffens, *The Shame of the Cities* (New York: McClure, Phillips & Co., 1904; reprint ed., New York: Hill & Wang, 1968), p. 4.

9. Rothman examines the single institution of the Senate and professionalization in *Politics and Power*, pp. 1–8, 126, and 137–48.

10. William L. Riordan. ed., *Plunkitt of Tammany Hall* (New York: E. P. Dutton & Co., 1963), pp. 17 and 19.

11. "Politics as a Vocation" and "Science as a Vocation," in *From Max Weber: Essays in Sociology*, trans. and ed. H. H. Gerth and C. Wright Mills (New York: Oxford University Press, 1958), pp. 110–11 and 137.

12. John J. Beer and W. David Lewis, "Aspects of the Professionalization of Science," in *The Professions in America*, pp. 110–30; and A. Hunter

Dupree, *Science in the Federal Government: A History of Policies and Activities to 1940* (Cambridge, Mass.: Belknap Press of Harvard University Press, 1957), pp. 169–73.

13. Wilbur J. Cash, *The Mind of the South* (New York: A. A. Knopf, 1941; reprint ed., New York: Vintage Books, 1969), pp. 250–59; C. Vann Woodward, *Origins of the New South, 1877–1913* (Baton Rouge: Louisiana State University Press, 1971), pp. 369–95; Dewey W. Grantham, Jr., *The Democratic South* (Athens: University of Georgia Press, 1963), pp. 1–14 and 42–68; and William C. Havard, ed., *The Changing Politics of the South* (Baton Rouge: Louisiana State University Press, 1973), pp. 3–36.

14. W. Richard Scott. "Professionals in Bureaucracies—Areas of Conflict," in *Professionalization*, ed. Howard M. Vollmer and Donald L. Mills (Englewood Cliffs, N.J.: Prentice-Hall, 1966), pp. 270–74.

15. Robert H. Wiebe, *The Search for Order, 1877–1920* (New York: Hill & Wang, 1967), pp. 111–32; see also Charles S. Hyneman, *Bureaucracy in a Democracy* (New York: Harper, 1950); Joseph La Palombara, ed., *Bureaucracy and Political Development* (Princeton, N.J.: Princeton University Press, 1963); Martin Albrow, *Bureaucracy* (New York: Praeger, 1970); Norman John Powell, *Responsible Public Bureaucracy in the United States* (Boston, Mass.: Allyn & Bacon, 1967); Francis E. Rourke, ed., *Bureaucratic Power in National Politics* (Boston, Mass.: Little, Brown, 1965); and Peter M. Blau and Marshall W. Meyer, *Bureaucracy in Modern Society*, 2d ed. (New York: Random House, 1971).

CHAPTER 2

1. Susan Brown Lyon to the author, 19 December 1968; interview with Col. Campbell Brown, Nashville, Tenn., 5 August 1968; William T. Hale and Dixon L. Merritt, *A History of Tennessee and Tennesseans: The Leaders and Representative Men in Commerce, Industry and Modern Activities*, 4 vols. (Chicago & New York: Lewis Publishing Co., 1913), 4:938–39; Albert Nelson Marquis, ed., *Who's Who in America*, vol. 8 (Chicago: A. N. Marquis Co., 1914–15), p. 298; and *Nashville Tennessean*, 5 August 1935.

2. Interview with Susan Brown Lyon, Murfreesboro, Tenn., 26 January 1973; the Lucius Polk Brown Papers, James D. Hoskins Library, University of Tennessee, Knoxville, include letters and receipts dealing with George Campbell Brown's stockbreeding activities.

3. Linda Arret, Alderman Library, University of Virginia, to the author, 23 March 1973; Certificates of Completed Courses, Lucius Polk Brown Papers, Tennessee State Library and Archives, Nashville; Progress Report to George Campbell Brown, 1 December 1886, in the possession of Lucia Brown Brownell, Birmingham, Ala.

4. George Campbell Brown to Lucius Polk Brown, 26 February 1889, Brown Papers, University of Tennessee, box 3-A, is typical of this correspondence.
5. Tennessee Agricultural Experiment Station, *Second Annual Report, 1889* (Knoxville: n.p., 1890), pp. 1–2 and 9–11; *Third Annual Report, 1890* (Knoxville: n.p. 1891), pp. 10–11.
6. M. A. Scovell to Lucius Polk Brown, 6 January 1891, Brown Papers, University of Tennessee, box 2-B.
7. William Waller, ed., *Nashville in the 1890s* (Nashville, Tenn.: Vanderbilt University Press, 1970), pp. vii–viii, 3–15, 118, and 120.
8. Marquis, *Who's Who in America*, 8:298; interview, Susan Brown Lyon.
9. Marquis, *Who's Who in America*, 8:298; interview, Susan Brown Lyon; William O. Batts, Jr., registrar, Vanderbilt University, to the author, 1 March 1973; Lucius P. Brown, "The Phosphate-Rock Deposits of Tennessee," *Engineering Magazine* 12 (October 1896–March 1897): 86–100; interview with Col. Campbell Brown, Franklin, Tenn., 27 January 1973.
10. Interview, Susan Brown Lyon; *Lynchburg (Virginia) News*, 15 December 1903.
11. Brown to Gov. James B. Frazier, 14 January 1903, and Edward Ward Carmack to Frazier, 13 January 1903, Gov. James B. Frazier Papers, Tennesse State Library and Archives, Nashville, box 25, file 2; Robert M. Allen to Frazier, 27 June 1903, box 6, file 2; Brown to Frazier, 30 July 1903, box 6, file 5; and National Association of State Dairy and Food Departments, *Proceedings of the Eighth Annual Convention, 1904* (n.p.: National Association of State Dairy and Food Departments, 1904), p. 54. The name of this organization changed slightly over the years; alterations will be reflected in the text and notes.
12. Carl Bridenbaugh, *Cities in Revolt: Urban Life in America, 1743–1776* (New York: Knopf, 1955), pp. 28–32 and 98; Blake, *Public Health in Boston*, pp. 14–16; Richard C. Wade, *The Urban Frontier: The Rise of Western Cities, 1790–1830* (Cambridge, Mass.: Harvard University Press, 1959), pp. 80, 84, and 98–99; Rosenberg, *Cholera Years*, pp. 40, 133, and 210–24; Robert Ernst, *Immigrant Life in New York City, 1825–1863* (Port Washington, N.J.: I. J. Friedman, 1965), pp. 28–29; Wilson G. Smillie, *Public Health Administration in the United States* (New York: Mac-Millan, 1935), pp. 11–12; Richard Harrison Shryock, *Medicine and Society in America, 1660–1860* (New York: New York University Press, 1960), pp. 117–66; Roy Lubove, *The Progressives and the Slums: Tenement House Reform in New York City, 1890–1917* (Pittsburgh, Pa.: University of Pittsburgh, 1962), pp. 12–25; Charles-Edward A. Winslow, *The Evolution and Significance of the Modern Public Health Campaign* (New Haven, Conn.: Yale University Press, 1933), pp. 28–35; and Howard D. Kramer, "Effect of the Civil War on the Public Health Movement," *Mississippi Valley Historical Review* 35 (December 1948): 449–62.

13. Gerald M. Capers, Jr., "Yellow Fever in Memphis in the 1870's," *Mississippi Valley Historical Review* 24 (March 1938): 485–86.

14. Ibid., pp. 490-96; see also John M. Keating, *A History of the Yellow Fever: The Yellow Fever Epidemic of 1878, in Memphis, Tennessee* (Memphis, Tenn.: Howard Association, 1879); and William D. Miller, *Memphis during the Progressive Era, 1900–1917* (Memphis, Tenn.: Memphis State University Press, 1957), p. 113.

15. F. Garvin Davenport, "Scientific Interests in Kentucky and Tennessee, 1870–1890," *Journal of Southern History* 14 (November 1948): 509; John E. Windrow, *John Berrien Lindsley, Educator, Physician, Social Philosopher* (Chapel Hill: University of North Carolina Press, 1938), pp. 113–63.

16. Joseph C. Kiger, "Social Thought as Voiced in Rural Middle Tennessee Newspapers, 1878–1898," *Tennessee Historical Quarterly* 9 (June 1950): 143.

17. George E. Waring, Jr., "The Cleaning of a Great City," *McClure's,* September 1897, p. 912.

18. Richard Hofstadter, "Beard and the Constitution: The History of an Idea," *American Quarterly* 2 (Fall 1950): 208.

19. Interview with Thomas Ripley Bryant, director of Agricultural Extension Work, retired, Kentucky Agricultural Experiment Station, Lexington, 9 March 1973.

20. Walter Lippmann, *Drift and Mastery: An Attempt to Diagnose the Current Unrest* (New York: Mitchell Kennerley, 1914; Englewood Cliffs, N.J.: Prentice-Hall, 1961), p. 53; Thomas D. Clark, *Pills, Petticoats, and Plows: The Southern Country Store* (Indianapolis, Ind., and New York: Bobbs-Merrill Co., 1944), pp. 192–208; and Young, *Toadstool Millionaires.*

21. Mark Sullivan, *Our Times: The United States, 1900–1925,* vol. 1: *The Turn of the Century* (New York: Charles Scribner's Sons, 1926), pp. 590–91; and Anderson, *Health of a Nation,* provides a comprehensive study of Wiley's career.

22. Association of State and National Food and Dairy Departments, *Proceedings of the Eleventh Annual Convention, 1907* (New York: John Wiley & Sons, 1908), p.[2].

23. National Association of State Dairy and Food Departments, *Proceedings of the Sixth Annual Convention, 1902* (n.p.: National Association of State Dairy and Food Departments, 1903), p. 337.

24. Tennessee, 51st Assembly, 1899, *Appendix to House and Senate Journals,* p. 426.

25. Tennessee, 51st Assembly, 1899, *House Journal,* pp. 71, 82, 363, and 503; 334, 366, and 534; and 589, 609, and 976; 52d Assembly, 1901, *House Journal,* pp. 154, 166, 473, and 549; 194, 217, 462, 469, and 732; 215, 231, and 732; and 284, 297, and 452; 53rd Assembly, 1903, *House Journal,* pp. 304 and 606; 53rd Assembly, 1903, *Senate Journal,* p. 339; 54th

Assembly, 1905, *House Journal*, pp. 431, 454, and 542; and 460, 491, and 713.

26. Tennessee, *Revised Statutes, Annotated* (Nashville: Shannon, 1917), 1:2812.
27. *Nashville Banner*, 16 and 22 January 1907.
28. Tennessee, 55th Assembly, 1907, *House Journal*, pp. 118–19.
29. Ibid., p. 478; *Nashville Banner*, 29 January, 4, 5, 6, and 15 February, and 6, 21, and 28 March 1907.
30. *Nashville Banner*, 28 March and 4 and 10 April 1907; Tennessee, 55th Assembly, 1907, *Senate Journal*, p. 608.
31. Tennessee, *Revised Statutes*, 1:2812–19.
32. *Nashville Tennessean*, 6 January 1908.
33. Diary, 2 and 7 January 1908, Brown Papers, Nashville.
34. Diary, 9–15 January 1908; interview, Campbell Brown, 5 August 1968.

CHAPTER 3

1. Stanley J. Folmsbee, Robert E. Corlew, and Enoch L. Mitchell, *Tennessee: A Short History* (Knoxville: University of Tennessee Press, 1969). pp. 422–33.
2. U.S., Department of Commerce, Bureau of the Census, *Thirteenth Census of the United States, 1910: Population*, 3:739.
3. Pure Food and Drug Inspector's Report, 1908, p. 17, Gov. Malcolm R. Patterson Papers, Tennessee State Library and Archives, Nashville, box 2, file 3; Pure Food and Drug Inspector's Report, 1914, p. 13, Gov. Ben W. Hooper Papers, Tennessee State Library and Archives, Nashville, box 12, file 3. All official reports of the pure food and drug inspector cited hereinafter are included in governors' papers, all of which are located at the state library and archives.
4. Charles V. Chapin, *A Report on State Public Health Work, Based on a Survey of State Boards of Health* (Chicago: American Medical Association, 1916), p. 52.
5. National Association of State Dairy and Food Departments, *Proceedings of the Sixth Annual Convention*, 1902, p. 397.
6. Pure Food and Drug Inspector's Report, 1908, pp. 2–3 and 17; Brown, "Report of the State Pure Food and Drug Inspector, January 25, 1909," in Tennessee, Board of Health, *Biennial Report of the State Board of Health of Tennessee from January, 1907 to January, 1909* (Nashville: Foster & Parkes Co., 1909), pp. 267–68 and 279.
7. Diary, 18 January, 19 February, and 6 March 1908.
8. Diary, 1, 8, and 16 October 1908; interview, Campbell Brown, 27 January 1973.
9. *Chattanooga Daily Times*, 12 December 1908.

10. Diary, 15 January 1908; *Nashville Tennessean*, 17 and 20 March and 8 April 1908.
11. *Nashville Tennessean*, 9 February 1909.
12. Brown, "Report to the State Board of Health, January 25, 1909," pp. 276–77.
13. *Nashville Tennessean*, 12 December 1908.
14. *Nashville Tennessean*, 25 October 1908.
15. Brown, "Report to the State Board of Health, January 25, 1909," p. 25.
16. Diary, 17 January and 29 September 1908; interview, Campbell Brown, 27 January 1973.
17. *Nashville Tennessean*, 5 May 1909.
18. Nashville Housekeepers' Club to Brown, 27 November 1908, and Nashville Board of Trade to Brown, 28 December 1908, Brown Papers, Nashville.
19. Tennessee, 56th Assembly, 1909, *House Journal*, pp. 397, 671, and 759; *Senate Journal*, p. 789; and Brown, "Report to the State Board of Health, January 25, 1909," pp. 272–73.
20. *Nashville Tennessean*, 5 May 1909.
21. Brown, *Bulletin Number 3*, included in "Report of the State Pure Food and Drug Inspector, October 4, 1910," in Tennessee, Board of Health, *Biennial Report of the State Board of Health from January, 1909 to January, 1911* (Nashville: Foster & Parkes Co., 1911), p. 126; Pure Food and Drug Inspector's Report, 1910, pp. 3–4, Patterson Papers, box 2, file 3.
22. *Nashville Tennessean*, 12 May 1909.
23. *Nashville Banner*, 14 May 1909.
24. *Nashville Tennessean*, 7 July 1909.
25. *Nashville Tennessean and American*, 6 April and 9, 11, and 25 July 1911.
26. *Nashville Tennessean and American*, 16 September 1911.
27. Pure Food and Drug Inspector's Report, 1909, pp. 2–3, Patterson Papers, box 2, file 3.
28. *Memphis Commercial-Appeal*, 18 April 1912, and *Nashville Tennessean and American*, 20 April 1912.
29. These statistics were taken from the annual reports of the pure food and drug inspector.
30. Pure Food and Drug Inspector's Report, 1913, p. 3, Hooper Papers, box 12, file 4.
31. Brown, "Report to the State Board of Health, January 25, 1909," p. 294; and *Nashville Tennessean and American*, 6 April 1911.
32. Pure Food and Drug Inspector's Report, 1909, p. 3; *Nashville Tennessean*, 26 May and 20 August 1909.
33. Pure Food and Drug Inspector's Report, 1909, pp. 2–3; Pure Food and Drug Inspector's Report, 1912, pp. 6–7, Hooper Papers, box 12, file 3.
34. Kentucky, Agricultural Experiment Station, *Twentieth Annual Report, 1907* (Lexington: n.p., 1907), p. xiv.

35. Brown, "Report of the State Pure Food and Drug Inspector, April 8, 1910," in Tennessee, Board of Health, *Biennial Report*, p. 39.
36. Ibid., p. 40; *Nashville Tennessean*, 20 September 1910.
37. Brown, *Bulletin Number 3*, p. 94.
38. Ibid., pp. 149–50.
39. Brown, "What the Pure Food and Drug Laws Do for the Farmer," in Tennessee, Department of Agriculture, *Biennial Report of the Department of Agriculture, 1909–1910* (Nashville: Brandon Printing Co., 1911), pp. 365–68.
40. Ibid., p. 372.
41. Brown, *Bulletin Number 3*, p. 117.
42. Pure Food and Drug Inspector's Report, 1908, pp. 10–14, and 1909, p. 1.
43. Ibid., 1909, p. 1, and 1912, p. 5.
44. Ibid., 1910, p. 5; and *Nashville Tennessean and American*, 27 December 1911.
45. "Report to the State Board of Health, April 8, 1910," p. 37; and Pure Food and Drug Inspector's Report, 1910, p. 1.
46. Pure Food and Drug Inspector's Report, 1910, p. 6; and *Nashville Tennessean and American*, 9 July 1911.
47. Brown to Wiley, 29 September 1909, and Wiley to Brown, 18 October 1909, Wiley Papers, Library of Congress, Manuscripts Division, Washington, D.C., container 74.
48. Anderson, *Health of a Nation*, pp. 210–11.
49. Ibid., p. 214.
50. Ibid., pp. 229–31; *Nashville Tennessean*, 29 August 1909.
51. Pure Food and Drug Inspector's Report, 1909, pp. 3–4.
52. Brown to Mrs. Harvey W. Wiley, 7 May 1912, Wiley Papers, container 108.
53. Association of State and National Food and Dairy Departments, *Proceedings of the Fourteenth Annual Convention, 1910* (n.p.: Association of State and National Food and Dairy Departments, 1910), p. 192; idem, *Proceedings of the Fifteenth Annual Convention, 1911* (n.p.: Association of State and National Food and Dairy Departments, 1911), p. 108.
54. Anderson, *Health of a Nation*, pp. 244–47; see also Anderson, "The Pure-Food Issue: A Republican Dilemma, 1906–1912," *American Historical Review* 61 (April 1956): 550–73.
55. Association of State and National Food and Dairy Departments, *Proceedings of the Fifteenth Annual Convention*, pp. 108–9; and Robert M. Allen to Wiley, 29 July 1912, Wiley Papers, container 109.
56. *Nashville Tennessean and American*, 26 August 1911.

CHAPTER 4

1. Thomas B. Alexander, *Political Reconstruction in Tennessee* (Nashville,

Tenn.: Vanderbilt University Press, 1950), pp. 11–225; James Welch Patton, *Unionism and Reconstruction in Tennessee, 1860–1869* (Chapel Hill: University of North Carolina Press, 1934), pp. 51–123 and 201–41.

2. Daniel Merritt Robison, *Bob Taylor and the Agrarian Revolt in Tennessee* (Chapel Hill: University of North Carolina Press, 1935), pp. 14–16; a newer, different interpretation can be found in Roger L. Hart, *Redeemers, Bourbons & Populists: Tennessee, 1870–1896* (Baton Rouge: Louisiana State University Press, 1975).

3. Paul E. Isaac, *Prohibition and Politics: Turbulent Decades in Tennessee, 1885–1920* (Knoxville: University of Tennessee Press, 1965), pp. 10–11.

4. Ibid., pp. 32–98 and 116–29.

5. Ibid., pp. 137–58; Eric Russell Lacy, "Tennessee Teetotalism: Social Forces and the Politics of Progressivism," *Tennessee Historical Quarterly* 24 (Fall 1965): 219–40; Stanley J. Folmsbee, Robert E. Corlew, and Enoch L. Mitchell, *History of Tennessee*, 4 vols. (New York: Lewis Publishing Co., 1960), 2:216–24.

6. Folmsbee et al., *History of Tennessee*, 2:216–24.

7. Diary, 15, 21 and 22 January 1908; reappointment, 23 November 1909, Brown Papers, Nashville.

8. *Nashville Tennessean and American*, 31 May and 28 June 1911.

9. *Nashville Tennessean and American*, 2 and 7 December 1911.

10. *Nashville Tennessean and American*, 7 December 1911; *Nashville Banner*, 8 December 1911.

11. *Nashville Tennessean and American*, 28 December 1911; Association of American Dairy, Food and Drug Officials, *Proceedings of the Sixteenth Annual Convention, 1912* (n.p.: Association of American Dairy, Food and Drug Officials, 1912), p. 15.

12. *Nashville Tennessean and American*, 27 December 1911 and 7 January 1912; interview, Campbell Brown, 5 August 1968.

13. Wiley to Ben W. Hooper, 18 September 1911; Wiley to Brown, 18 September 1911; Brown to Wiley, 21 September 1911, Wiley Papers, container 94.

14. Brown to Wiley, 27 December 1911; Wiley to Brown, 3 January 1912, Wiley Papers, container 110.

15. *Nashville Tennessean and American*, 7 December 1911.

16. *Nashville Tennessean and American*, 13 December 1911 and 6 January 1912.

17. *Nashville Tennessean and American*, 13 December 1911.

18. *Nashville Tennessean and American*, 13 December 1911.

19. *Nashville Tennessean and American*, 13 December 1911.

20. *Nashville Tennessean and American*, 14 January 1912.

21. *Nashville Tennessean and American*, 5 January 1912; *Nashville Banner*, 2 January 1912.

22. *Nashville Banner*, 10 January 1912.

23. *Nashville Tennessean and American*, 15 January 1912.
24. *Nashville Tennessean and American*, 16 January 1912.
25. *Nashville Tennessean and American*, 18 and 19 January 1912; *Nashville Banner*, 16 January 1912.
26. *Nashville Tennessean and American*, 16 January 1912.
27. *Nashville Tennessean and American*, 2 March 1912; *Nashville Banner*, 1 March 1912.
28. *Knoxville Daily Journal and Tribune*, 6 January 1912; *Nashville Tennessean and American* (quoting the *Knoxville Sentinel*), 11 January 1912; *Chattanooga Daily Times*, 12 December 1908; *Memphis Commercial-Appeal*, 2 March 1912.
29. *Nashville Tennessean and American*, 13 December 1911 and 14 January 1912.
30. Isaac, *Prohibition anl Politics*, p. 104.
31. Everett Robert Boyce, ed., *The Unwanted Boy: The Autobiography of Governor Ben W. Hooper* (Knoxville: University of Tennessee Press, 1963), p. 85. Hooper was illegitimate, a fact he readily admitted. He holds the distinction of being the only known governor of Tennessee to admit publicly that he was a bastard.
32. *Nashville Tennessean and American* (quoting *Washington Times*), 17 March 1912, and 18 March 1912.
33. *Nashville Tennessean and American*, 30 March, 21 July, and 8 December 1912.
34. *Nashville Tennessean and American*, 20 and 26 April, 2 and 26 May, and 11 July 1912; *Memphis Commercial-Appeal*, 18 April 1912; Pure Food and Drug Inspector's Report, 1912, pp. 2–16; Association of American Dairy, Food and Drug officials, *Proceedings of the Sixteenth Annual Convention*, p. 18.
35. *Nashville Tennessean and American*, 2 November 1912.

CHAPTER 5

1. Pure Food and Drug Inspector's Report to Special Legislative Committee, 12 March 1913, pp. 1–6, Hooper Papers, box 12, file 3.
2. Tennessee, 58th Assembly, 1913, *House Journal*, p. 68.
3. Isaac, *Prohibition and Politics*, pp. 218–19; Brown to Wiley, 1 July 1913, Wiley Papers, container 111.
4. *Nashville Tennessean and American*, 5 January and 14 and 21 September 1913; Report to Legislative Committee, p. 8.
5. "Weekly Chats with Consumers," 6 June 1914, Brown Papers, Nashville.
6. S. W. Stratton to Hooper, 15 January 1913; Hooper to Stratton, 21 January 1913; and Hooper's secretary to Stratton, 1 May 1913, Hooper Papers, box 6, file 5.
7. *Nashville Tennessean and American*, 8 February 1915.

8. *Nashville Tennessean and American*, 5 October 1913; W. W. Draper to Hooper (n.d.), 1912; Hooper to Draper, 5 March 1912, Hooper Papers, boxes 3 and 13, file 13.
9. Diary, 19 and 23 March 1915.
10. *Nashville Tennessean and American*, 14 February 1914; Pure Food and Drug Inspector's Report, 1913, p. 5.
11. "Weekly Chats with Consumers."
12. *Nashville Tennessean and American*, 5 October 1913, and 11 January and 29 March 1914; Pure Food and Drug Inspector's Report, 1914, p. 10.
13. Lucius P. Brown, "Enforcement of the Tennessee Anti-Narcotics Law," *American Journal of Public Health* 5 (April 1915): 323.
14. Ibid.
15. *Nashville Tennessean and American*, 3 March and 3 April 1914; *Hyde v. State*, 131 Tenn. 208–20 (1914); Theodore J. McMorrough to J. A. Rafferty, 13 May 1915, Brown Papers, Nashville.
16. *Memphis Press*, 6 April 1914; and Pure Food and Drug Inspector's Report, 1914, pp. 4–5.
17. Brown, "Enforcement of the Tennessee Anti-Narcotics Law," pp. 326–31.
18. Ibid.
19. Musto, *American Disease*, pp. 97–102 and passim.
20. Brown, "Enforcement of the Tennessee Anti-Narcotics Law," p. 333.
21. Diary, 18, 19, and 20 January 1915; John S. Akin to Brown, 21 May 1915, and James B. Newman to Brown, 15 May 1915, Brown Papers, Nashville.
22. Interview, Susan Brown Lyon.
23. Isaac, *Prohibition and Politics*, pp. 232–39.
24. Tennessee, 59th Assembly, 1915, *House Journal*, pp. 146–47.
25. *Nashville Tennessean and American*, 18 June 1915.
26. Interview, Susan Brown Lyon.
27. Diary, 26 and 30 April and 3 May 1915.
28. Interview, Susan Brown Lyon; New York City, Board of Health, *Annual Report, 1915* (New York: Board of Health, 1916), List of the Medical Advisory Board; Edwin R. Lewinson, *John Purroy Mitchel: The Boy Mayor of New York* (New York: Astra Books, 1965), pp. 81–82; and Brown to Susan Massie Brown, 15 August 1915, Brown Papers in the possession of his daughter Susan Brown Lyon, Murfreesboro, Tenn. Hereinafter, these letters will be cited as Brown to wife, with the appropriate date. Also, all Brown Papers dealing with his work in New York City are in Murfreesboro.
29. *New York Times*, 18 May 1915; *Nashville Tennessean and American*, 18 May 1915; Diary, 3 May 1915; Robert Belcher to Brown, 5 May 1915; Brown to Dr. S. S. Goldwater, 20 May 1915; and Brown to Fort, 4 June 1915, Brown Papers, Nashville; interview, Susan Brown Lyon.
30. These letters and telegrams are contained in the Brown Papers, Nashville; Anonymous to Brown, 18 May 1915.

31. Brown to wife, 22 June 1915.
32. Brown to wife, 25 June 1915.
33. Brown to wife, 30 June 1915.
34. Numerous applications and endorsements are included in the Gov. Tom C. Rye Papers, box 58, file 1; *Nashville Tennessean and American*, 19 July 1915; *Knoxville Sentinel*, 15 June 1915.
35. *Nashville Tennessean and American*, 13, 14, and 25 July 1915.
36. *Nashville Tennessean and American*, 12 and 18 July 1915; *Nashville Banner*, 10 July 1915; H. P. Fritz to Rye, 13 July 1915, and William Hall to Rye, 13 July 1915, Rye Papers, box 58, file 1.
37. *Nashville Tennessean and American*, 18 July 1915.
38. *Nashville Tennessean and American*, 23 July 1915.
39. *Nashville Tennessean and American*, 26 July 1915; *Nashville Banner*, 26 July 1915; and Brown to wife, 1 August 1915.

Chapter 6

1. *Thirteenth Census*, 3:187 and 739. The following sources are useful in understanding the plight of the immigrants as viewed by reformers: Robert W. De Forest and Lawrence Veiller, eds., *The Tenement House Problem*, 2 vols. (New York: MacMillan, 1903); Robert Hunter, *Poverty* (New York: MacMillan, 1912); and John Spargo, *The Bitter Cry of the Children* (New York: MacMillan, 1906). Roy Lubove and Bayrd Still provide historical perspective on the immigrants in New York. See Lubove, *Progressives and the Slums*, and Still, *Mirror for Gotham: New York as Seen by Contemporaries from Dutch Days to the Present* (New York: New York University Press, 1956), pp. 205–56.
2. Brown to wife, 25 June 1915.
3. Brown to wife, 15 August 1915.
4. Brown to wife, 15 August 1915.
5. Brown to wife, 20 September 1915.
6. Charles F. Bolduan, *Over a Century of Health Administration in New York City* (New York: Department of Health, March 1916), pp. 13–15; see also Gordon Atkins, *Health, Housing, and Poverty in New York City, 1865–1898* (Ann Arbor, Mich.: Edwards Brothers, 1947), p. 34; Lubove, *Progressives and the Slums*, pp. 12–25.
7. Bolduan, *Over a Century of Health Administration*, pp. 18–27; Wallace S. Sayre and Herbert Kaufman, *Governing New York City: Politics in the Metropolis* (New York: W. W. Norton, 1965), pp. 11–17; and John A. Krout, "Framing the Charter," in *The Greater City: New York, 1898–1948*, ed. Allan Nevins and John A. Krout (New York: Columbia University Press, 1948), pp. 41–60.
8. Sayre and Kaufman, *Governing New York City*, p. 97; memorandum, 28

May 1957, Department of Health of the City of New York, Haven Emerson Public Health Library, New York City.

9. Bolduan, *Over a Century of Health Administration*, p. 31; New York City, Board of Health, *Annual Report*, *1914* (New York: Board of Health, 1915), p. 25. Hereinafter annual reports will be cited as such with appropriate dates and pages.

10. Brown to wife, 3 August 1915.

11. *Annual Report, 1915*, pp. 22 and 36.

12. Bolduan, *Over a Century of Health Administration*, p. 21; Atkins, *Health, Housing, and Poverty*, pp. 150–55.

13. Bolduan, *Over a Century of Health Administration*, pp. 31 and 33; and *Annual Report, 1915*, p. 71.

14. *New York Times*, 22 November 1916; and *Annual Report, 1917*, p. 46.

15. Brown to wife, 1 August 1915; and New York City, Board of Health, *Staff News* (New York: Board of Health, 1 July 1915), 3:3; *Staff News* (1 February 1916), 4:5. Hereinafter this publication will be cited by title with appropriate volume, date, and page.

16. *Annual Report, 1916*, p. 68; *New York Times*, 27 May 1916.

17. *New York Times*, 27, 28, and 30 May 1916.

18. Notes on employees, 1918, Brown Papers.

19. Brown to wife, 9 and 17 July 1915; and undated clipping from the *New York Globe and Commercial Advertiser*, Brown Papers.

20. New York City, Board of Health, *Weekly Bulletin*, new ser. (New York: Board of Health, 25 December 1915), 4: 413–14; *Annual Report, 1916*, p. 70.

21. Brown to wife, 5 August 1915.

22. *Staff News* (1 November 1915), 3:5; (1 January 1916), 4:5–6; (1 April 1917), 5:4; and (1 June 1917), 5:3.

23. *Annual Report, 1915*, p. 74.

24. Unidentified clipping, Brown Papers.

25. *New York Times*, 1 September 1915.

26. *Annual Report, 1915*, pp. 75–76.

27. *New York Times*, 5 October 1915.

28. Brown, "Healthy Food Handlers," *Monthly Bulletin* (New York: Board of Health, November 1915), 5:277–79; "Restaurants and Disease," *Outlook*, 12 January 1916, pp. 59–60; *New York Times*, 30 May 1916; and *New York Tribune*, 13 June 1916.

29. *New York Times*, 6 and 7 June 1916.

30. *New York Times*, 9 and 15 June 1916.

31. *New York Times*, 16, 17, 20, and 21 June and 24 July 1916; and *Annual Report, 1916*, pp. 24–25. From June to November, there were 8,991 cases of poliomyelitis reported, resulting in 2,448 deaths.

32. *Annual Report, 1916*, p. 25; and *New York Times*, 31 January and 25 March 1917.

33. Laura A. Cauble, "Clean Food for City Dwellers," *American City*, July 1916, pp. 18–21; and *Annual Report, 1915*, pp. 77 and 83.
34. Lawrence Veiller, "Housing and Health," *The Public Health Movement*, included in *Annals of the American Academy of Political and Social Science*, vol. 37, no. 2 (March 1911), p. 18.
35. Donald B. Armstrong, "Educational Work in Sanitary Food Values in New York City," *American Journal of Public Health* 5 (April 1915): 349–50; M. E. Ravage, "My Plunge into the Slums," *Harper's Magazine*, April 1917, p. 660; and *Annual Report, 1915*, p. 77.
36. "How New York Is Fed," *Scribner's Monthly*, October 1877, pp. 729–30.
37. *Annual Report, 1915*, p. 76.
38. *New York Times*, 25 July 1916.
39. *Annual Report, 1915*, pp. 82–83; *Annual Report, 1916*, p. 74.
40. *Annual Report, 1916*, pp. 68–69; *Annual Report, 1917*, p. 46; and *New York Times*, 19 and 28 December 1915, 2 January 1916, and 14 July 1917. The Sanitary Code was amended eventually, and by 1919, patent-medicine manufacturers were registering the contents of their products.
41. *New York Times*, 18 May and 2 July 1917.
42. John Purroy Mitchel to Mrs. W. B. Meloney, 20 July 1917, John Purroy Mitchel Papers, Library of Congress, Manuscripts Division, Washington, D.C., container 13.
43. *Annual Report, 1917*, p. 44; Mabel H. Kittredge, "Food Salvage in New York," *New Republic*, 11 August 1917, pp. 43–45; Lucius P. Brown, "Partial Analysis of Food-Waste Problem," *Journal of Home Economics* 9 (November 1917): 503–4; "Food Conservation in New York City," *Annals of the American Academy of Political and Social Science* 74 (November 1917): 140–46; "Food Wastes—Some Causes and Remedies," *Journal of the Franklin Institute* 185 (May 1918): 585–610; and "Practical Aspects of Dehydrated Foods," *American Journal of Public Health* 8 (May 1918): 372–73.
44. Brown to wife, 6 and 8 September 1915; Lucius P. Brown, "The Experience of New York City in Grading Market Milk," *American Journal of Public Health* 6 (July 1916): 671–77; and brief prepared for Brown's Defense, 1918, pp. 91, 93, and 94, Brown Papers.
45. Brief, p. 91; *New York Times*, 28 September 1916; *Staff News* (1 September 1916), 4:5. See also Lucius P. Brown and Clarence V. Ekroth, "Relation of the Fat in Milk to the Solids-Not-Fat," *Journal of Industrial and Engineering Chemistry* 9 (March 1917): 297–99; in the same issue, "Chemical Quality of New York City Market Milk," pp. 299–301.

CHAPTER 7

1. Arnold S. Rosenberg, "The New York Reformers of 1914: A Profile," *New York History* 50 (April 1969): 187–206.

2. *Boston Transcript*, 25 May 1916, clipping included in the Mitchel Papers, Library of Congress, container 10.

3. Haven Emerson, "A Health Program for New York City," *Collected Works of Haven Emerson*, Haven Emerson Public Health Library, New York City (typewritten).

4. S. S. Goldwater to the Editors of the *New York Times*, *World*, *Herald*, *Tribune*, *Sun*, and *Post*, 17 September 1917, Mitchel Papers, Library of Congress, container 10.

5. Haven Emerson to S. L. Martin, 31 March 1917, Mayor John Purroy Mitchel Papers, Municipal Archives and Records Center, New York City, container 235.

6. David Craig Ringsmuth, "The Mayor of New York City: A Study of Growth in Responsibility, Authority and Resources" (Ph.D. diss., Columbia University, 1970), pp. 160–61; Lewinson, *John Purroy Mitchel*, pp. 18–95.

7. Lewinson, *John Purroy Mitchel*, pp. 95–103.

8. Ibid., p. 239.

9. Ibid., p. 149; and Gustavus Myers, *The History of Tammany Hall*, 2d ed., rev. and enl. (New York: Boni & Liveright, Inc., 1917; reprint ed., New York: Burt Franklin, 1968), pp. 399–400.

10. William L. Chenery, "So This Is Tammany Hall!" *Atlantic Monthly*, September 1924, pp. 311 and 319.

11. J. Joseph Huthmacher, "Boss Murphy and Progressive Reform," in *Urban Bosses, Machines, and Progressive Reformers*, ed. Bruce M. Stave (Lexington, Mass.: D. C. Heath & Co., 1972), pp. 92–98; Weiss, *Charles Francis Murphy*; "Murphy, Chieftain," *Outlook*, 7 May 1924, pp. 10–11; and Richard Barry, "Mr. Murphy—the Politicians' Politician," *Outlook*, 14 May 1924, p. 54.

12. Anna Lanahan, "The Attempt of Tammany Hall to Dominate the Brooklyn Democratic Party: 1903–1909" (M.A. thesis, Columbia University, 1955), pp. 69–71; Lewinson, *John Purroy Mitchel*, p. 213.

13. Alfred Connable and Edward Silberfarb, *Tigers of Tammany: Nine Men Who Ran New York* (New York: Holt, Rinehart & Winston, 1967), pp. 259–60.

14. Ringsmuth, "The Mayor of New York," p. 164; and "New York's Mayor-Elect a Self-Made Man," *Literary Digest*, 17 November 1917, pp. 46–48. See also John F. Hylan, *Mayor Hylan of New York: An Autobiography* (New York: Rotary Press, 1922), and William Bullock, "Hylan," *American Mercury*, April 1924, p. 449.

15. Lewinson, *John Purroy Mitchel*, pp. 214–30; and Melvyn Dubofsky, "Success and Failure of Socialism in New York City, 1900–1918: A Case Study," *Labor History* 9 (Fall 1968): 361–75.

16. *Brooklyn Daily Eagle*, 23 September 1917, clipping included in the Mitchel Papers, Library of Congress, container 15.

17. "New York's Return to Tammany," *Literary Digest*, 17 November 1917, p. 13. See also Eda Amberg and William H. Allen, *Civic Lessons from Mayor Mitchel's Defeat* (New York: Institute for Public Service, 1921).

18. *New York World*, 7 November 1917; *New York Globe*, 7 November 1917; *New York Post*, 7 November 1917; *New York American*, 7 and 10 November 1917; all of these clippings are contained in Scrapbook, vol. 14, Edwin P. Kilroe Collection of Tammaniana, Columbia University's Butler Library, Special Collections, New York City.

19. *New York World*, 16 and 28 November 1917; *New York Times*, 17 and 24 November 1917; *New York Post*, 20 and 28 November 1917; *New York Tribune*, 28 November 1917; and *New York American*, 28 November 1917, vol. 14, Kilroe Collection.

20. *New York Times*, 2 December 1917.

21. *New York Times*, 6 December 1917.

22. *New York Times*, 8 January 1918; *New York Tribune*, 22 January 1918; and *New York World*, 21 January 1918, vol. 14, Kilroe Collection.

23. *New York Times*, 16 January and 10 April 1918.

24. *New York Times*, 10 April 1918.

25. *New York Times*, 13 April 1918.

26. Charles A. Beard, "Human Nature and Administration," *Nation*, 25 April 1918, pp. 503–4.

27. *New York Times*, 13 and 16 April 1918.

28. *New York Times*, 11, 12, and 13 April 1918.

29. *New York Times*, 12 April 1918; and *New York Herald*, 14 April 1918.

30. *New York Herald*, 17 April 1918; *New York Times*, 16 and 17 April 1918.

31. *New York Times*, 25, 26, and 29 April 1918; *New York Herald*, 25 April 1918; and unidentified clipping, Brown Papers.

32. *New York Times*, 18, 22, and 30 April 1918; John F. Hylan to J. Lewis Amster, 29 April 1918, Mayor John F. Hylan Papers, Municipal Archives and Records Center, New York City, location 418.

33. Taxpayer to Hylan, n.d., received 19 April 1918, and anonymous letter to Copeland, n.d., received 4 May 1918, Senator Royal S. Copeland Papers, Michigan Historical Collections, University of Michigan, Ann Arbor, box 11.

34. *New York Times*, 17 and 21 April 1918.

35. *New York Times*, 1 May 1918; *New York Evening Sun*, 30 April 1918, the latter contained in vol. 14, Kilroe Collection.

36. *New York Times*, 27 and 28 April 1918; *New York Herald*, 8 May 1918; and interview, Susan Brown Lyon.

37. *New York Times*, 30 April 1918; *New York Globe and Commercial Advertiser*, 6 May 1918; *Brooklyn Daily Eagle*, 8 May 1918; *Who Was Who in America* (Chicago: A. N. Marquis Co., 1950), 1:259–60.

38. Unsigned letter to Copeland, 6 May 1918, Copeland Papers, box 10.

39. *New York Times*, 1 May 1918; *New York Herald*, 2 May 1918.

40. *New York Times,* 1 and 2 May 1918.
41. *Staff News,* 1 May 1918, 6:1.
42. *New York Sun,* 3 May 1918; *New York Times,* 3 and 5 May 1918; and Copeland to Charles D. Howard, 24 May 1918, Brown Papers.
43. Carl E. McCombs to Lillian D. Wald, 15 May 1918, Lillian D. Wald Papers, Columbia University's Butler Library, Special Collections, New York City, box 90.
44. Brief, pp. 1–11.
45. *New York Times,* 11 May 1918; editorial, "Retrogression in New York City," *Journal of the American Medical Association* 70 (27 April 1918): 1231; editorial, "The New York Health Department," *Journal of the American Medical Association* 70 (25 May 1918): 1539; and A. W. Hedrich to Brown, 15 July 1918, Brown Papers.
46. Brief, pp. 35–36 and 41–44; Wiley to Brown, 29 June 1918; Brown to Dr. William C. Woodward, 31 May 1918; and Robert M. Allen to Charles D. Howard, 2 July 1918, Brown Papers.
47. *New York World,* 5 June 1918.
48. Tom C. Rye to Brown, 24 June 1918, Rye Papers, box 33, file 3; brief, pp. 39–40 and 45–46; James B. Frazier to Brown, 2 July 1918, Brown Papers; and *Nashville Tennessean and American,* 28 April, 3 and 27 May, 9 June, 2 and 14 July, and 11 August 1918.
49. *New York Times,* 29 May 1918.
50. *New York Times,* 30 May 1918.
51. *New York Times,* 2 June 1918; and Brown to Copeland, 10 June 1918, Brown Papers.
52. Brown to Copeland, 10 June 1918; and *New York Times,* 12 June 1918.
53. Interview, Col. Campbell Brown, 27 January 1973; and brief.
54. *New York Times,* 6 July 1918; and Brown to Board of Health, n.d., Brown Papers.
55. *New York American,* 11 August 1918; and *New York Tribune,* 11 August 1918.
56. Alice Lakey to Brown, 10 July 1918, and Brown to Lakey, 16 July 1918, Brown Papers.
57. Connable and Silberfarb, *Tigers of Tammany,* pp. 265–66.
58. *New York Times,* 17 November 1927.
59. *New York Times,* 18 and 19 September 1918; "The Hylan Administration," *Searchlight,* 30 October 1918, pp. 11–12, contained in the Brown Papers; *The ABC of Hylanism* (New York: n.p., 1925), Citizens Union Papers, Columbia University's Butler Library, Special Collections, New York City, box A-20; see also John F. Hylan, *Seven Years of Progress, 1918–1925,* Report to the Board of Aldermen (New York: n.p., 1925).
60. *New York Times,* 1 and 2 February 1923; *Annual Report, 1926,* pp. 5–6.
61. *New York Herald,* 8 June 1918; *New York Times,* 7 May and 17 August

1918; 11, 12, 13, 14, 15, 19, 20, 21, 24, 25, and 27 January, and 2 February 1919.

CHAPTER 8

1. Jackson, *Food and Drug Legislation in the New Deal*, pp. 3–23; and Young, *Medical Messiahs*, pp. 158–59.
2. Vernon L. Parrington, *Main Currents in American Thought: An Interpretation of American Literature from the Beginnings to 1920*, vol. 3: *The Beginnings of Critical Realism in America, 1860–1920* (New York: Harcourt, Brace & World, 1958), p. 412; and Allen F. Davis, *Spearheads for Reform: The Social Settlements and the Progressive Movement, 1890–1914* (New York: Oxford University Press, 1967), pp. 222 and 227.
3. See Richard Hofstadter, *The Age of Reform: From Bryan to F. D. R.* (New York: Knopf, 1955); George E. Mowry, "The California Progressive and His Rationale: A Study in Middle Class Politics," *Mississippi Valley Historical Review* 36 (September 1949): 239–50; Robert H. Wiebe, *Businessmen and Reform: A Study of the Progressive Movement* (Cambridge, Mass.: Harvard University Press, 1962); Gabriel Kolko, *The Triumph of Conservatism: A Reinterpretation of American History, 1900–1916* (New York: Free Press of Glencoe, 1963); J. Joseph Huthmacher, "Urban Liberalism and the Age of Reform," *Mississippi Valley Historical Review* 49 (September 1962): 231–41; Samuel P. Hays, "The Politics of Reform in Municipal Government in the Progressive Era," *Pacific Northwest Quarterly* 55 (October 1965): 157–69; Keith L. Bryant, Jr., "Kate Barnard, Organized Labor and Social Justice in Oklahoma during the Progressive Era," *Journal of Southern History* 35 (May 1969): 145–64.
4. Parrington, *Beginnings of Critical Realism*, p. 403.
5. Brown to Copeland, 30 September 1918, Brown Papers.
6. John F. Murlin to Brown, 20 July 1918; Brown to Murlin, 5 August 1918; and Brown to Casper W. Miller, 6 August 1918. All Brown Papers related to his military service are in Murfreesboro.
7. Brown to Miller, 26 August 1918; Murlin to Brown, 28 August 1918; and Brown to Murlin, 30 August 1918, Brown Papers.
8. *New York Evening Post*, 1 October 1918, and an unidentified clipping, Brown Papers; Lucia Brown Brownell, daughter of Lucius Polk Brown, to author, 17 July 1973.
9. U.S., Army, Surgeon General, *The Medical Department of the United States Army in the World War* (Washington, D.C.: U.S. Government Printing Office, 1926–27), 1:74.
10. M. N. Baker, "The Municipal Health Program," *National Municipal Review* 2 (April 1913): 200-209; J. L. Rice, "A City Health Officer Looks at Public Health," *American Journal of Public Health* 31 (November

1941): 1121–27; W. C. Rucker, "Progam of Public Health for Cities," *American Journal of Public Health* 7 (March 1917): 228; and Charles-Edward A. Winslow, "The Untilled Fields of Public Health," *Science* 51 (9 January 1920): 30.

11. *Medical Department of the U.S. Army in the World War*, 1:74.

12. Ibid., pp. 308 and 540.

13. Ibid.. pp. 308–9; and U.S., Department of War, Office of the Surgeon General, *Annual Reports, 1918*, 1:693.

14. U.S., Department of War, Office of the Surgeon General, *Annual Reports, 1919*, 1:2741; Charles H. Collins, *Conservation of Food in the United States Army, 1917–1919* (Typescript), Army War College Historical Section Study no. 37 (1943), p. 29.

15. *Medical Department of the U.S. Army in the World War*, 1:311–12.

16. Collins, *Conservation of Food in the U.S. Army*, pp. 50–51.

17. Inspection forms for use of mess officers, Camp Bowie, Texas, 15 January 1919; Capt. Lucius P. Brown to Camp Bowie Executive Officer, 27 December 1918; Capt. Lucius P. Brown to Commanding General, Hoboken, New Jersey, 16 June 1919; Discharge, 19 July 1919; and Brown to D. C. Absger, Executive Officer, 396th Medical Regiment, 81st Division, Knoxville, Tennessee, 23 February 1924. All of this correspondence is contained in the Brown Papers.

18. Brown to Copeland, 23 September 1919, and Copeland to Brown, 26 September 1919, Brown Papers.

19 Copeland to Brown, 26 September 1919, Brown Papers. This memorandum is not the same as the one cited above, but another communication written the same day.

20. Copeland to directors of bureau, 21 July 1919; and Copeland to Brown, 4 October 1919, Brown Papers. See also Jackson, *Food and Drug Legislation in the New Deal*, p. 92.

21. Brown to Frank J. Monaghan, 9 October 1919, Brown Papers.

22. *New York Times*, 1 March 1919; *Annual Report, 1919*, pp. 193–94; New York State, Department of Narcotic Control, "Special Rules and Regulations for the City of New York," Brown Papers; and Musto, *American Disease*, pp. 156–63.

23. Numerous communications regarding these summons appear in the Brown Papers; New York City, Criminal Courts, *Record of Indictments*, 11:48 and 64.

24. Resignation, 27 December 1920, Brown Papers.

25. *Nashville Tennessean and American*, 28 December 1919; *Nashville Banner*, 27 December 1919; and *Nashville Tennessean*, 1 January 1920.

26. Association of American Dairy, Food and Drug Officials, *Proceedings of the Sixteenth Annual Convention, 1912*, pp. 16 and 18; Burton J. Hendrick, "The Farce of the Pure Food Law," *McClure's*, August 1914, pp. 77–87;

and Hendrick, "Eight Years of the Pure Food Law," *McClure's*, March 1915, pp. 59–70 and 138–42.

27. Lucia Brown Brownell to author; interview, Susan Brown Lyon; and Robert J. Bassett, reference librarian at the University of Tennessee, to Edith Keys, reference librarian at East Tennessee State University, 11 March 1974. Bassett secured information concerning the Merrell-Soule Company from William Alonzo Stocking, *Manual of Milk Products* (New York: MacMillan, 1917).

28. Interview, Susan Brown Lyon; and Lizinka Brown Mosley, daughter of Lucius Polk Brown, to author, 20 June 1973.

29. Interview, Susan Brown Lyon; and Brown to Lucia Cabell Brown, 20 May 1925, in the possession of Lucia Brown Brownell, Birmingham, Ala.

30. Interview, Susan Brown Lyon; Lizinka Brown Mosley to author; and Lucia Brown Brownell to author.

31. Lucia Brown Brownell to author.

32. *Nashville Banner*, 28 November 1929, clipping in possession of Lucia Brown Brownell; invitations to White House Conference, Brown Papers, Nashville; and White House Conference, *Directory of Committee Personnel, July 1, 1930*, Library of Congress, Washington, D.C.

33. "The Copeland Bill," *Nation*, 28 March 1934, p. 344; Connable and Silberfarb, *Tigers of Tammany*, pp. 259–60; editorial, "The Copeland Bill," *American Journal of Public Health* 25 (August 1935): 961–62; editorial, "Federal Legislation to Control Foods, Drugs, and Cosmetics: The Copeland Bill," *American Journal of Public Health* 27 (April 1937): 381–83; W. S. Frisbie, "Public Health Aspects of the Federal Food, Drug, and Cosmetic Act," *American Journal of Public Health* 29 (December 1939): 1292–96; and interview with Mrs. Llewellyn H. King, personal secretary to Sen. Royal S. Copeland, Murfreesboro, Tenn., 26 January 1973.

34. Brown to Oswald Garrison Villard, 25 April 1934; and Brown to James Rorty, 13 September 1934, in the possession of Lucia Brown Brownell.

35. Lucia Brown Brownell to author; interview, Susan Brown Lyon.

36. Brown to Mark Granite, 21 January 1935, in the possession of Lucia Brown Brownell.

37. Interview, Susan Brown Lyon; *Nashville Banner*, 5 April 1935.

Index

named an official of United States Bureau of Weights and Measures, 33; uses campaign technique in Tennessee, 33–37; seeks additional appropriations, 41; appoints special agents, 42; addresses American Chemical Society, 43; elected to vice-presidency and presidency of national food and drug organization, 44, 45–46, 54, 80; position of, on food additives, 44–45; influence of Tennessee politics on, 48, 51; reappointed by Patterson, 51; reappointment conflict of, 51–61; opposition to, 52–53; works against false weights and measures, 52, 53; adopts grading system, 52, 53; supporters of, 53, 55, 56, 57, 60–61; his opinion of Hooper, 54; answers charges, 57–58; reappointed by Hooper, 58; supported for chief chemist of United States Department of Agriculture, 61; addresses food officials, 62; traces growth of department, 66; as superintendent of weights and measures, 67; his supervision of Tennessee employees, 67–68; enforces Sanitary Hotel Law, 69; enforces Anti-Narcotics Act, 69, 70–72; in court, 70, 72; addresses American Public Health Association, 71–72; and enforcement of the liquor laws, 74; applies for directorship in New York City, 74; accepts New York City appointment, 76; and employees in New York City, 76–77; describes New York City tenement districts, 83–84; harbors misgivings about New York City position, 84–85; has faith in New York City civil service, 88; defines responsibilities, 89; becomes acquainted with employees, 90–91; his involvement in public health education,

92–93; seeks good relations with businessmen, 93; uses campaign technique, 94; takes up "the raid," 94–95; scrutinizes fish business, 95; adopts grading system, 96; campaigns against exposed food, 98–99; supports conservation, 101; professional activities of, 102; initial work of, in New York City compared to Tennessee, 102–3; as target of politicians, 104; is called before Civil Service Commission, 114; decides to fight Tammany, 119; attacked by MacBride, 120; accusations against, and his denial of, 120; suspended by Copeland, 121; prepares defense, 121; responds to charges, 122; supported by professional groups and friends, 122–23; requests extension of hearing date, 124; questions Copeland's motives, 124–25; submits brief at hearing, 125; is reinstated, 126; demonstrates difficulty of removing civil-service appointee, 128; is only director vindicated of charges, 130; life of, altered by New York City health controversy, 131; enters Sanitary Corps, 133; returns to New York City position, 138; his controversy with Copeland, 138–40; resigns New York City position, 140; experience of, as food and drug official disillusioning, 140; takes dim view of enforcement under Pure Food and Drug Act, 1906, 141; returns to Tennessee, 142; as promotion agent for Merrell-Soule Company, 142; as administrator general of American Dairy Products Company, 142; attends White House Conference on Child Health and Protection, 143; and Copeland bill, 144; death of, 145; as product of and molder of